YEAR BOOK OF
CARDIOLO
Heart

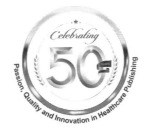

Celebrating 50 Years

Passion, Quality and Innovation in Healthcare Publishing

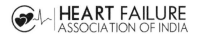
HEART FAILURE
ASSOCIATION OF INDIA

YEAR BOOK OF CARDIOLOGY – 2019
Heart Failure

Chief Editor

Vijay K Chopra MD DM FACC FESC FHFA

Director
Heart Failure Program
Medanta – The Medicity
Gurugram, Haryana, India

Forewords

Stefan D Anker

Inder S Anand

JAYPEE BROTHERS MEDICAL PUBLISHERS
The Health Sciences Publisher
New Delhi | London

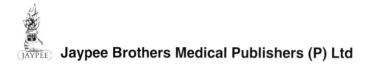

Jaypee Brothers Medical Publishers (P) Ltd

Headquarters

Jaypee Brothers Medical Publishers (P) Ltd
4838/24, Ansari Road, Daryaganj
New Delhi 110 002, India
Phone: +91-11-43574357
Fax: +91-11-43574314
Email: jaypee@jaypeebrothers.com

Overseas Offices

J.P. Medical Ltd
83 Victoria Street, London
SW1H 0HW (UK)
Phone: +44 20 3170 8910
Fax: +44 (0)20 3008 6180
Email: info@jpmedpub.com

Website: www.jaypeebrothers.com
Website: www.jaypeedigital.com

Year Book of Cardiology – 2019 Heart Failure / *Vijay K Chopra*

First Edition: **2019**

ISBN: 978-93-5270-894-9

Printed at: Sterling Graphics Pvt. Ltd. India.

CONTRIBUTORS

Chief Editor

Vijay K Chopra MD DM FACC FESC FHFA
Director
Heart Failure Program
Medanta – The Medicity
Gurugram, Haryana, India

Contributing Authors

Abraham Oomman MD DM DNB MNAMS FACC
FSCAI
Senior Consultant
Interventional Cardiology, Apollo Hospital
Chennai, Tamil Nadu, India

Balbir Singh MD DM FACC
Chairman
Division of Electrophysiology
Department of Cardiology
Medanta – The Medicity
Gurugram, Haryana, India

Bhagirath Raghuraman MD DNB DM (Cardiology)
Senior Consultant Cardiology
Program Director, Heart Transplant
Narayana Institute of Cardiac Sciences
Narayana Health City
Bengaluru, Karnataka, India

Hari Krishnan MBBS MD DM DNB (Cardiology)
Professor of Cardiology
Sree Chitra Tirunal Institute for
Medical Sciences and Technology
Thiruvananthapuram, Kerala, India

Jagdish Chander Mohan MBBS MD DM MNAMS
FASE
Consultant Emeritus
Fortis Hospital Shalimar Bagh and
Chairman of Institute of Heart and
Vascular Disease, Jaipur Golden Hospital
New Delhi, India

K Venugopal MBBS MD DM
Professor and Head
Department of Cardiology
Pushpagiri Institute of Medical Sciences
and Research Centre
Thiruvalla, Kerala, India

Madhu Shukla MBBS Dip Card (London) PhD
Consultant
Non Invasive Cardiology, Jaipur Golden Hospital
New Delhi, India

Sandeep Seth DM Cardiology
Professor Cardiology
All India Institute of Medical Sciences
New Delhi, India

Tihirugnanasambandan Sunder MS FRCS (Eng)
FRCS (Cardiothoracic) FCCP (USA)
Senior Consultant Cardiothoracic and
Heart-Lung Transplant Surgeon, Apollo Hospitals
Chennai, Tamil Nadu, India

Uday Jadhav MD FACC FAHA FSCC FRCP FICC
FCSI
Cardiology Department
MGM New Bombay Hospital
Navi Mumbai, Maharashtra, India

Vishwas Mohan MBBS Dip Card (London) PhD
Associate Consultant
Max Patparganj Hospital
New Delhi, India

FOREWORD

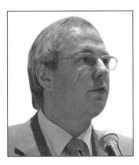

Stefan D Anker MD PhD FESC
Professor
Department of Innovative Clinical Trials
University Medical Center Göttingen
Göttingen, Germany

Over the last decade, I am keenly interested in the progress, in the attention and care for heart failure patients in India. This process was accompanied by a great advancement in academic exchange and communication in and on heart failure. The process was lead by the Heart Failure Association of India in a most laudable way. As President of the Heart Failure Association of the ESC and later as its Past-President, I repeatedly had the chance to first-hand experience of their work at many conferences. Heart failure—particularly chronic heart failure—is a great place of progress of cardiovascular medicine in the same time span with new drugs and devices coming to the forefront of clinical medicine in reality. The book on heart failure we have now in our hands is attempting to give an executive summary of these developments by highlighting important papers and giving commentary that helps the reader for context. This format will aid the cardiologist of today, always keen to learn more, but also short on time. I wish the HFAI's new *Year Book of Cardiology – 2019 Heart Failure* all the success of the world. I am sure that the interested reader will get the knowledge needed to refine his/her care for the growing number of heart failure patients that need it.

FOREWORD

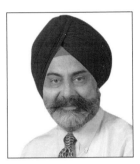

Inder S Anand MD FRCP D Phil (Oxon)
Professor of Medicine
University of Minnesota Medical School
VA Medical Center Minneapolis MN and
San Diego, California, USA

It is extremely heartening to notice the remarkable progress, Indian Cardiology community has made in embracing the importance of the management of heart failure, during the last decade. This is reflected in the large number of meetings dedicated to heart failure, attendance at these meetings and the rapidity at which heart failure clinics are growing in the country. At the last meeting of the Heart Failure Association of India (HFAI), held in New Delhi in February 2019, the leadership of the HFAI decided that to further the interest of heart failure in the country, efforts be made to circulate to its members, in a digestible form, some of the most important recent publication on heart failure at regular intervals.

The publication of the first *Year book of Heart Failure 2017* containing important publication in the field during the last year is a landmark achievement. Dr Chopra and all the other authors are to be congratulated for gathering so much information in one volume. The book has several chapters edited by some of India's leading and distinguished investigators and clinicians. They have done a remarkable job in collecting the most outstanding publications with the highest impact on a number of diverse topics including basic science research, heart failure registries, advances in management of treatment of chronic and acute decompensated heart failure. All readers, and particularly the busy clinician will find the format of providing the abstract of the publications followed by a brief commentary extremely helpful.

The book will be extremely useful to the cardiovascular specialist and internist caring for the growing number of these patients. It will be equally helpful to the scientists and the trainees. The readers will eagerly await the next year's Yearbook.

PREFACE

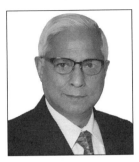

Vijay K Chopra MD DM FACC FESC FHFA
Director
Heart Failure Program
Medanta – The Medicity
Gurugram, Haryana, India

Heart failure has witnessed some remarkable new developments over the past few years. The literature is vast, and it becomes difficult to keep up with all that has been happening, be it basic research, diagnostics, available therapeutics or techniques under development. This small handbook by the Heart Failure Association of India is an attempt to give a snapshot of the most important developments in this field. The book is divided into 9 Sections, each containing a brief summary of the best articles in that field followed by comments from an expert. The period covered is from April'18 to March'19. I do hope you find it useful. Your comments and suggestions will be very welcome to make this yearly publication better in future.

I would like to sincerely thank all the contributors of this handbook for their diligence in finding the best articles and giving their valuable insights.

CONTENTS

Section 3: Registries

Section Editor: Hari Krishnan

Section 4: Biomarkers

Section Editor: Uday Jadhav

Section 5: Imaging in Heart Failure in 2018

Section Editors: Jagdish Chander Mohan, Madhu Shukla, Vishwas Mohan

Section 6: Acute Heart Failure

Section Editors: K Venugopal, Vijay K Chopra

Section 7: Chronic Heart Failure

Section Editors: Abraham Oomman, Vijay K Chopra

Section 8: Electrophysiology, Pacing and Ablation

Section Editor: Balbir Singh

Section 9: Left Ventricular Assist Device and Transplant

Section Editor: Thirugnanasambandan Sunder

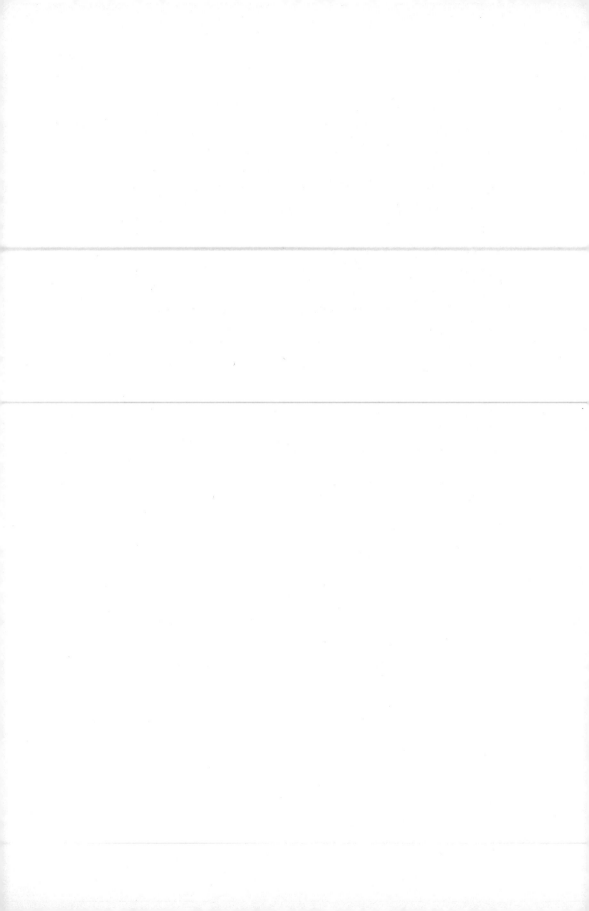

PLATE 1

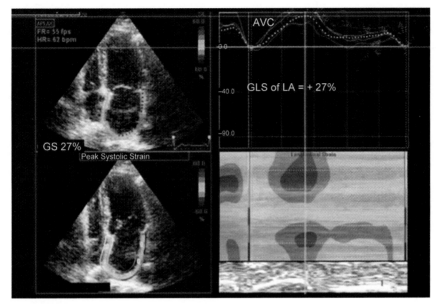

(GLS: global longitudinal strain)

FIG. 5: Peak global left atrial (LA) longitudinal strain of +27% in a patient with heart failure with reduced ejection fraction (HFrEF). *(Chapter 5)*

Section 1

Basic Sciences

Section Editor: Bhagirath Raghuraman

Biomarkers for the Identification of Cardiac Fibroblast and Myofibroblast Cells

Tarbit E, Singh I, Peart JN, et al. Biomarkers for the identification of cardiac fibroblast and myofibroblast cells. *Heart Fail Rev. 2019;24(1):1-15.*

*Abstract**

In heart repair and function, the importance of cardiac fibroblast and myofibroblast cells has been recognized by several experimental researches. In normal healthy heart, there is a central role of the cardiac fibroblast in the electrical, chemical, and structural aspects within the heart. It is interesting to note that in the development of heart failure, transformation of the cardiac fibroblast cells to the cardiac myofibroblast cells is thought to play an important part. It is always a challenge to differentiate between the two cells types. As myofibroblast cells are expressed only in failing or stressed heart, therefore, a better understanding of the cell function can aid in identifying therapies that help in the repair of damaged heart. This article will give an outline of what is presently known regarding the physiological and pathological roles within the heart, cardiac fibroblasts, and myofibroblasts; their pathological and physiological roles within the heart; and the causes of the transition of fibroblasts into myoblasts. Potential markers that are available for characterizing these cells were also reviewed and it was observed that there is not a single cell-specific marker that delineates fibroblast cell or myofibroblast cell. Vimentin is commonly used for characterizing the cells of fibroblast origin. Discoidin domain receptor 2 (DDR2) is used to distinguish cardiac fibroblasts; whereas, myofibroblasts can be identified using α-smooth muscle actin. A known cytokine, transforming growth factor beta-1 (TGF-β1), is well known for causing transformation of the cardiac fibroblasts to the myofibroblasts. In this review, clinical treatments that can reduce or inhibit the actions of TGF-β1 along with its contribution to heart failure and cardiac fibrosis are also discussed.

> *"We need to identify potential cell-specific markers for cardiac fibroblast and myofibroblast cells, which will allow for new potential targets for the treatment of heart failure"*

COMMENT

The basic problem is that there is no single cell-specific marker exists, which delineates fibroblast cells or myofibroblast cells. By using discoidin domain receptor 2 (DDR2),

*Redrafted abstract

cardiac fibroblasts can be recognized; whereas, myofibroblasts can be identified using α-smooth muscle actin. Presently, periostin is evolving as a potential marker for myofibroblasts. A combination of presently available markers is recommended to be used for studying myofibroblasts and fibroblasts as accurately as possible. Implementing proteomics research in the future may help to identify cardiac biomarkers for heart failure (HF) and would enable a more tailored treatment approach. It is well known that transforming growth factor beta-1 (TGF-β1) mediates the activation of fibroblast cells and their transformation to myofibroblasts and that both cell types have a contribution in fibrosis and impaired heart function.

Modifying TGF-β1 may pave the way to modulate HF. Cardiac fibroblast cells have no cell-specific marker for identification, and as a consequence, research within its field is often challenging. Under various conditions, cardiac fibroblasts may be triggered to transform into the myofibroblast cells. There is a major requirement to identify the potential cell-specific markers for cardiac fibroblast and myofibroblast cells that will allow for new potential targets in the treatment of HF. Most of the current available treatment targets that are available for cardiac fibrosis/HF are broad-acting; these are not recommended for long-term use because they can affect the quality of life of patient because of unwanted side effects. In the future, microRNA-130a and TGF-β have potential as new targets in treatment of HF and cardiac fibrosis. However, there is need for further research to be conducted.

────(**Key Message**)────

⊙ *Most of the therapeutic options currently available for cardiac fibrosis/HF are broad-acting and not recommended because they can have an impact on the quality of life of the patient by causing unwanted side effects. The microRNA-130a and TGF-β have potential as new targets in treatment of heart failure and cardiac fibrosis in the future.*

ARTICLE 2

Advances in the Diagnosis and Treatment of Transthyretin Amyloidosis with Cardiac Involvement

Rigopoulos AG, Ali M, Abate E, et al. Advances in the diagnosis and treatment of transthyretin amyloidosis with cardiac involvement.
Heart Fail Rev. 2019;24(4):521-33.

Abstract*

Amyloidosis is caused due to extracellular deposition of insoluble abnormal fibrils made by misfolded proteins that can modify the anatomy of tissues and impede the function of various

*Redrafted abstract

organs including the heart. Amyloidosis affecting the heart comprises transthyretin amyloidosis (ATTR) and systemic amyloidosis (amyloid light chain, AL). The former can be acquired among elderly patients [wild-type transthyretin (ATTRwt)] or can be inherited among younger individuals [mutant transthyretin (ATTRm)]. The diagnosis is required given that the high phenotypic heterogeneity of disease. Thus, "red flags" are extremely valuable as they are suggestive features that give support to diagnostic suspicion. The lack of broad awareness in clinicians, however, is a significant barrier to early diagnosis and treatment of ATTR. Additionally, the need for endomyocardial biopsy (EMB) has been revisited by latest implementation of noninvasive diagnostic techniques. While AL amyloidosis needs tissue confirmation and typing for diagnosis, ATTR can presently be diagnosed noninvasively by combination of bone scintigraphy and absence of monoclonal protein. Securing the correct diagnosis is crucial for the newly available therapeutic options that target both ATTRm and ATTRwt and are either directed at stabilizing the abnormal protein or at reducing transthyretin production. This article is aimed at reviewing contemporary aspects of the diagnosis and management of transthyretin amyloidosis with cardiac involvement and summarizing the latest therapeutic advances with patisiran, tafamidis and inotersen.

"Amyloidosis undoubtedly is one of the most challenging clinical conditions to treat, especially because it involves uncontrolled deposition of structurally abnormal proteins (amyloid fibrils) in multiple organs, such as the liver, kidney, eyes, nervous system, gastrointestinal tract, and the heart, which increase the patients' morbidity and mortality"

COMMENT

This article comprehensively assesses the magnitude of the problem of amyloidosis. To sum up, amyloidosis includes uncontrolled deposition of the structurally abnormal proteins (i.e. amyloid fibrils), which affects multiple organs, like the eyes, kidney, liver, nervous system, heart, and gastrointestinal tract, and eventually increases the morbidity and mortality of patients. More than 30 different amyloidogenic proteins have been recognized. The immunoglobulin light-chain amyloidosis (AL) and the transthyretin amyloidosis (ATTR) are two most common types of amyloidosis; the latter constitutes the mutant transthyretin (ATTRm) and the wild-type transthyretin (ATTRwt) entities. Patients can present with many nonspecific clinical signs and symptoms, which require a high clinical suspicion for early diagnosis along with laboratory findings, electrocardiography, multimodality imaging, and eventually biopsy diagnostics and genetic testing.

The treatment of amyloidosis has evolved from a situation of helplessness to a potentially curable condition. The promising new medications available today include tafamidis (Vyndaqel®), patisiran [given IV, it is a double-stranded synthetic oligonucleotide interfering with the RNA production of the abnormal transthyretin (TTR)], and inotersen (Tegsedi®) that is a single-stranded antisense oligonucleotide inhibitor of mutant and wild-type human TTR.

⊙ *The treatment of amyloidosis has evolved from a situation of hopelessness to a potentially curable condition. The promising new medications available today include tafamidis (Vyndaqel®), patisiran (given IV, it is a double-stranded synthetic oligonucleotide that interferes with the RNA production of the abnormal TTR), and inotersen (Tegsedi®) that is a single-stranded antisense oligonucleotide inhibitor of wild-type and mutant human TTR.*

(**Key Message**)

ARTICLE 3

Anti-apoptosis in Nonmyocytes and Pro-autophagy in Cardiomyocytes: Two Strategies against Postinfarction Heart Failure through Regulation of Cell Death/Degeneration

Takemura G, Kanamori H, Okada H, et al. Anti-apoptosis in nonmyocytes and pro-autophagy in cardiomyocytes: Two strategies against postinfarction heart failure through regulation of cell death/degeneration. *Heart Fail Rev. 2018;23(5):759-72.*

*Abstract**

For prevention or treatment of heart failure, antiapoptotic therapy for cardiomyocytes can be an effective strategy. To note, morphological evidence that definitively demonstrate cardiomyocyte apoptosis are very rare in case of actual heart diseases like heart failure and acute myocardial infarction. In contrast, interstitial noncardiomyocytes like granulation tissue cells die through apoptosis to form scar tissue within the postinfarction heart. Blockade of this apoptosis enhances survival and mitigates the ventricular remodeling and dysfunction in the chronic stage. For explaining this benefit, possible mechanisms might be preservation of the infarcted wall thickness along with preservation of the myofibroblasts that can promote infarct shrinkage; both will decrease the wall stress through Laplace law. Autophagy, on the other side, is an intracellular degradation mechanism that compensates for energy insufficiency by digesting and recycling intracellular components and is frequently observed in cardiomyocytes in failing heart with different roots including postinfarction. Autophagic degeneration in cardiomyocytes is strongly induced and activated by starvation. On inhibition of that activation, starved animals suffer with heart failure. Promotion of autophagy by several reagents or caloric restriction decreases the acute infarct size as well as mitigates the postinfarction cardiac remodeling and dysfunction in chronic stages. In addition, augmenting autophagy through treatment with exercise or resveratrol can

*Redrafted abstract

cause reverse remodeling among failing hearts with large old myocardial infarction. To conclude, two strategies are proposed to manage postinfarction heart failure through control of cell degeneration/death—antiapoptosis in granulation tissue noncardiomyocytes and proautophagy in salvaged cardiomyocytes.

"In the crusade against postinfarction heart failure, can we control or modify cell death or degeneration to alter the clinical course and outcome in such patients?"

COMMENT

Cell death and cell degeneration are not only related with the etiology of various heart diseases, but they are also clearly responsible for progression of those diseases. The end stage of many heart diseases is heart failure; among these diseases, most prevalent is ischemic heart disease. In heart failure, cell death is complicated due to existence of cross-talk among autophagy, apoptosis, and necrosis, sharing of certain signaling pathways, and exhibiting the same phenotypic morphological features in spite of various etiology and pathologic mechanisms. Apoptosis is a representative cell death modality; it presents with a very characteristic morphology, which can be clearly observed under an electron microscope. Cells that undergo apoptosis are shrunken and then fragmented along with an intact plasma membrane. Ultimately, they are consumed by neighboring cells like macrophages. Therefore, apoptotic cells do not push out their contents into the environment or cause inflammation. As a consequence, surrounding cells or interstitium are not damaged by them. For the worsening of heart failure, apoptotic cardiomyocyte death may be accountable; inhibition of this apoptosis can be used for prevention or treatment of heart failure. In this article, firstly, antiapoptotic therapy that targets granulation tissue nonmyocytes during the subacute stage of myocardial infarction has been described by the author. Subsequently, proautophagic therapy targeting cardiomyocytes in failing hearts is also described. We would recommend both approaches as new therapeutic strategies to mitigate heart failure by control of cell death and cell degeneration.

Key Message

⊙ *For worsening of heart failure, apoptotic cardiomyocyte death may be accountable; inhibition of apoptosis can be used for prevention or treatment of heart failure. Two strategies for management of postinfarction heart failure by controlling cell death and cell degeneration—(1) antiapoptosis in granulation tissue noncardiomyocytes; and (2) proautophagy in salvaged cardiomyocytes—are discussed elaborately in this article.*

ARTICLE 4

The Long Non-coding Road to Endogenous Cardiac Regeneration

Afify ARY. The long non-coding road to endogenous cardiac regeneration.
Heart Fail Rev. 2019;24(4):587-600.

Abstract*

A markedly low-regenerative capacity is possessed by human heart, which leaves patients with cardiac insults vulnerable to heart failure. This inability of regenerating lost myocardium is followed by comprehensive remodeling, resulting in further deterioration of cardiac functions and structure. Although the ability of regenerating in adult mammals seems to be lacking, some of the lower vertebrates possess cardioregenerative ability. Emerging studies disclosed that during development and soon after birth, mammals have the potential to undergo endogenous cardiac regeneration. It was later proved that the proliferation of the pre-existing cardiomyocyte pool is the source of the new cardiomyocytes. Currently, research is centered on discovering appropriate methods for restoring this lost potential in adulthood and improving cardiomyocyte proliferation ability. Long non-coding RNAs (lncRNAs) are critical functionally diverse epigenetic regulators that can either activate or repress gene expression. Previously, lncRNAs were involved in the cardiac development, lineage commitment, and aging. Recent studies indicate that lncRNAs possess capability of inducing endogenous cardiac regeneration by manipulation of gene expression in the cardiomyocytes. This review provides a brief overview of endogenous cardiac regeneration. It also summarizes and critically evaluates the present literature on lncRNAs' roles in endogenous cardiac regeneration and the difficulties facing in the field.

"A markedly low-regenerative capacity is possessed by human heart, which leaves patients with cardiac insults vulnerable to heart failure"

COMMENT

By regeneration of lost cardiomyocytes, it is expected that cardiac function and quality of life of heart failure (HF) patients are expected to improve. However, there is a requirement of comprehensive knowledge related to mechanisms and cellular pathways of cardiomyocytes for pursuing this hope. Two possible ways exist for achieving cardiac regeneration: (1) by supplying the myocardium exogenously with stem cells/cardiomyocytes that were originally reprogrammed from the nonmyocytes (i.e. cell therapy); and (2) by inducing endogenous regeneration from proliferation of the pre-existing cardiomyocyte pool. In recent studies, it has been shown that long non-coding RNAs (lncRNAs), a class of RNA molecules that lacks the capacity to translate into protein, play an enormous part in cardiac regeneration through their capacity to push

*Redrafted abstract

cardiomyocytes back into the cell cycle and allow them to proliferate and divide. The lncRNAs, therefore, represent new hope on the horizon for healing, failing hearts with the potential to induce cardiomyocyte regeneration.

Key Message

⊚ *Cardiac regeneration is achieved in two ways: (1) by supplying the myocardium exogenously with stem cells or cardiomyocytes; and (2) by inducing endogenous regeneration from proliferation of the pre-existing cardiomyocyte pool. Long non-coding RNAs (lncRNAs), a class of RNA molecules that lacks the capacity to translate into protein, play an enormous part in cardiac regeneration through their capacity to push cardiomyocytes back into the cell cycle and allow them to proliferate and divide.*

ARTICLE 5

Role of Cytokines and Inflammation in Heart Function During Health and Disease

Bartekova M, Radosinska J, Jelemensky M, et al. Role of cytokines and inflammation in heart function during health and disease.
Heart Fail Rev. 2018;23(5):733-58.

*Abstract**

Due to their actions on NF-κB, an inflammatory nuclear transcription factor, different cytokines have been reported to play significant regulatory roles in determination of cardiac function under physiological and pathophysiological conditions. Many cytokines comprising TNF-α, TGF-β, and various interleukins (like IL-1, IL-4, IL-6, IL-8 and IL-18) are implicated in development of several inflammatory cardiac pathologies, such as myocardial infarction, heart failure, cardiomyopathies, and ischemic heart disease. In case of ischemia-related pathologies, majority of the cytokines release into the circulation and serve as biological markers of inflammation. In addition, their direct role in the pathogenesis of ischemic injury is reported, which suggests that cytokines are potential targets for development of some of the anti-ischemic therapies. On the other side, some cytokines like IL-2, IL-4, IL-6, IL-8, and IL-10 are implicated in postischemic tissue repair and are therefore believed to have beneficial effects on cardiac function. Conflicting reports about the role of some cytokines in causing cardiac dysfunction in heart failure and distinct types of cardiomyopathy appear to be because of differences in the duration, degree, and nature of heart disease and the concentrations of some cytokines in circulation. No appropriate anticytokine treatment for enhancing cardiac function in any type of heart disease is accessible in the literature despite comprehensive studies in this field of investigation.

*Redrafted abstract

"It is well known that cytokines have been reported to play important regulatory roles in determination of cardiac function under both the physiological and the pathophysiological conditions. Can they be manipulated to modify cardiovascular disease outcomes?"

COMMENT

Cytokines mean "to set cells in motion"; a broad category of small proteins (approximately –30 kDa) is represented by them; they are also documented to serve as signaling molecules in regulating cellular function in both the health and the disease. These polypeptide factors, through paracrine, autocrine, and endocrine signal transduction mechanisms, have been proven to act as immunomodulatory agents. In particular, it has been shown that distinct cytokines have beneficial and deleterious impacts on cell function and are specifically implicated in inflammation, sepsis, and immune response, as well as trauma, reproduction, heart disease, and cancer. On the basis of their cell source, structure, or function, several cytokines are divided into different classes. However, this categorization is not absolute as each individual cytokine may belong to more than one class depending on its origin or structure. In particular, interferons, interleukins, and chemokines are included in these agents. It has been noted that cytokines have a significant impact on the cardiovascular system. Extensive study in this area has generated clear evidence that multiple cytokines including TNF-α and TGF-β and multiple interleukins are engaged in several heart pathological conditions like heart failure, acute myocardial infarction (AMI), and cardiomyopathies of different origins. The proinflammatory actions of TGF-β and TNF-α are mediated by the activation of NF-κB in cardiovascular disease (CVD). Proinflammatory cytokines, like IL-1 or IL-18, have been reported to play mostly negative roles in cardiac pathologies development and are proposed as potential targets for therapeutic interventions in the heart. Several cytokines, comprising IL-2, IL-4, and IL-6 with pleiotropic functions, appear to play a dual function in CVD and are suggested as markers of disease, including MI, as well as predictors of its adverse outputs. After acute damage to heart, some of these agents contribute in tissue repairing and are considered a therapeutic tool for heart disease treatment. To conclude, determining the exact role of any specific cytokines in the pathogenesis and progression of several types of CVD is a promising approach for developing novel therapeutic agents that target inflammatory processes implicated in disease processes in the heart. The establishment and implementation of anticytokine therapy as a standard treatment for heart disease is indeed a major challenge.

Key Message

⊙ *After acute damage to heart, some cytokines contribute in tissue repairing and are considered a therapeutic tool for heart disease treatment. It can be concluded that determining the exact role of any specific cytokines in the pathogenesis and progression of several types of CVD is a promising approach for developing novel therapeutic agents that target inflammatory processes implicated in disease processes in the heart and modifying the clinical outcomes.*

ARTICLE 6

Structural and Functional Abnormalities in Iron-depleted Heart

Kobak KA, Radwańska M, Dzięgała M, et al. Structural and functional abnormalities in iron-depleted heart. *Heart Fail Rev. 2019;24(2):269-77.*

*Abstract**

In heart failure (HF), iron deficiency (ID) is common and ominous comorbidity; it predicts worse outcomes regardless of the presence of anemia. Previous data from animal models of systemic ID indicate that ID is related to many structural and functional abnormalities of the heart. However, exact role of myocardial ID regardless of systemic ID and/or anemia is still unclear. In recent studies, for investigating the influence of ID on cardiac tissue, many transgenic models of cardiac-specific ID have been developed. In this review, structural and functional cardiac consequences of ID in these models have been discussed and data from clinical studies are summarized. Furthermore, useful effects of intravenous (IV) iron supplementation are described.

"We now have enough data to prove that ID is a common and ominous comorbidity in heart failure and predicts worse outcomes, regardless of presence of anemia. Treating this immensely treatable condition greatly alters clinical outcomes"

COMMENT

Focus of this review is on structural and functional abnormalities in heart as a result of systemic- or cardiac-specific iron deficiency (ID) along with strong emphasis on molecular evidence. One of the important microelements in body is iron because of its involvement in a variety of metabolic processes (such as transport of oxygen, synthesis of DNA, and oxidative energy production in electron transport chain). Iron is an essential component of Fe–S metalloproteins (key players in cellular energetics that can be found in the cytosol, mitochondria, and nucleus) in terms of its redox-based properties. The optimal iron supply is important especially for proper functioning of high-energy demand cells, particularly skeletal myocytes and cardiomyocytes. The most striking finding, however, was that intravenous iron therapy completely suppressed all morphological abnormalities and metabolic and contractile dysfunctions. It is well established that either iron overload or ID has an unfavorable effect on human condition and, in specific, in several papers, the role of disordered iron homeostasis in HF has been elucidated. Interestingly, all functional and morphological abnormalities were reversed by the supplementation of transferrin-bound iron. In addition, recent study has also shown that depletion of intracellular iron is harmful to cardiomyocyte and skeletal myocyte functioning and results in enhanced apoptosis and decreases cell viability.

*Redrafted abstract

(**Key Message**)

⊛ *Recent study demonstrates that depletion of intracellular iron is harmful to cardiomyocyte and skeletal myocyte functioning and leads to enhanced apoptosis and decreases the cell viability. Supplementation of transferrin-bound iron in heart failure greatly improves all morphological, metabolic, and contractile dysfunctions.*

ARTICLE 7

Metabolic Remodelling in Heart Failure

Bertero E, Maack C. Metabolic remodelling in heart failure.
Nat Rev Cardiol. 2018;15(8):457-70.

---

*Abstract**

Large amounts of energy are consumed by heart in form of ATP, which is continuously replenished in mitochondria by oxidative phosphorylation and, to a lesser extent, by glycolysis.

A complex network of enzymatic and signaling pathways regulates the metabolic flux of substrates toward their oxidation in mitochondria in order to adapt the ATP supply effectively to the constantly variable demand of cardiac myocytes. It is assumed that among heart failure patients, derangements of substrate utilization and intermediate metabolism, an energetic deficit, and oxidative stress underlie contractile dysfunction and disease progression. In this review, an overview of physiological processes of cardiac energy metabolism and their pathological alterations in diabetes mellitus and heart failure are provided. Though energetic deficit in failing hearts (which was discovered more than 2 decades ago) may account for the contractile dysfunction while maximal exertion, it is suggested that alterations of intermediate substrate metabolism and oxidative stress other than an ATP deficit as such account for the maladaptive cardiac remodeling and dysfunction under resting conditions. Treatments that target substrate utilization and/or oxidative stress in the mitochondria are presently being evaluated in heart failure patients and may be valuable tools in improving cardiac function beyond that attained by the neuroendocrine inhibition.

"Mitochondria play a big role in cardiac function and genesis of heart failure. Can their modulation alter disease processes and reverse or arrest the progress and onslaught of heart failure beyond that achieved by neuroendocrine inhibition?"

**Redrafted abstract

COMMENT

There is metabolic flexibility in healthy heart; it can derive energy from several circulating substrates. Heart failure (HF) is related with deranged substrate utilization, oxidative stress, and energy deficit. It is considered that these abnormalities contribute to the disease progression. HF is associated with derangements of all of the three fundamental steps of energy metabolism: (1) substrate uptake and utilization; (2) oxidative phosphorylation; and (3) energy shuttling through phosphotransfer systems. For cardiac ATP production, HF and diabetes mellitus are characterized by an enhanced reliance on the ketone bodies and fatty acid (FA) oxidation, respectively. It is a challenge to translate our understanding of these alterations into new therapeutic strategies due to intrinsic complexity of cardiac energy metabolism because the metabolic state of the heart is tightly intertwined with the elaborate network of signaling pathways and transcription factors that control gene expression. In this article, main features of cardiac energy metabolism in the healthy heart, its abnormalities in HF and (to a lesser extent) in diabetes mellitus, and the ultimate effects of metabolic derangement on cardiac structure and function are outlined. Rather than unbalanced substrate utilization, metabolic inflexibility and accumulation of toxic intermediates may detrimentally affect cardiac function. Metabolic intermediates can act as signaling factors, causing post-translational and epigenetic modifications or activating intracellular signaling cascades that eventually influence many cellular functions. The metabolism and excitation–contraction coupling derangements in the failing heart lead to mitochondrial dysfunction and oxidative stress. Targeting oxidative stress and/or metabolic alterations in mitochondria improves the development of HF in animal models, and translation of these approaches to HF patients is ongoing. The authors discuss options of treatment and if targeting substrate utilization and/or oxidative stress may improve cardiac function and enhance disease progression. The authors explained relevant question of whether altered substrate metabolism is a cause or a consequence of the contractile dysfunction in case of failing heart because this question is largely not answered. Indeed, it is suggested by experimental evidence that alteration in oxidative metabolism in mitochondria mainly associated with defective glucose and lactate oxidation precedes the cardiac dysfunction development, while increase in glycolytic activity and decrease in FA utilization are a result of the decline in oxidative metabolism. The ensuing mismatch between the FA uptake and the utilization may result in accumulation of the toxic lipid species, which possibly contributes to the HF progression. However, it is indicated by emerging evidence that myocardial metabolism in HF may become predominantly reliant on oxidation of ketone body, which possibly indicates an adaptive shift toward a more oxygen-efficient substrate. With respect to diabetes and HF, though both are characterized through different changes in the cardiac substrate metabolism, they finally lead to cytosolic accumulation of noxious metabolic intermediates. The authors also discuss those studies that show polarization of substrate utilization toward either FA or glucose is not adequate to cause glucotoxicity or lipotoxicity and, thus, is not detrimental as such. However, in case of pathological conditions, the shift toward a preferential substrate is related to accumulation of toxic intermediates and metabolic inflexibility, which might play dominant role in the cardiac dysfunction development and progression. Mitochondria appear to be abnormally clustered in the failing heart, and sarcoplasmic reticulum (SR)-mitochondria contact sites undergo structural reorganization that possibly impairs Ca^{2+} signaling between two organelles. Moreover, HF is characterized by derangements in excitation–contraction coupling, which negatively impacts the energy supply and demand matching in mitochondria. In failing cardiac myocytes, SR Ca^{2+} load and release are reduced, while trans-sarcolemmal NCX1-driven cytosolic Ca^{2+} influx is enhanced, both decrease the efficiency of mitochondrial Ca^{2+} uptake. In addition, intracellular Na^+ concentrations $[(Na^+)i]$ are increased in failing cardiac myocytes, which impair the mitochondrial Ca^{2+} accumulation during transitions of workload. The authors also discuss the evidence available for treatment options and explore the effects of the carnitine O-palmitoyltransferase 1 (CPT1A) inhibitor perhexiline and the metabolic modulator trimetazidine and the effects of sodium-glucose cotransporter-2 (SGLT-2; also known as SLC5A2) inhibitors among patients who had diabetes with high-cardiovascular risk.

(**Key Message**)

⊙ *Treatments that target oxidative stress and/or substrate utilization in mitochondria are presently being tested among patients who had heart failure and may be a promising tool in improving cardiac function beyond that attained by neuroendocrine inhibition. The authors also discuss the evidence available for treatment options and explore the evidence, effects, and benefits of treatment with perhexiline, trimetazidine, as well as SGLT-2 inhibitors.*

ARTICLE 8

The Relevance of microRNA in Post-infarction Left Ventricular Remodelling and Heart Failure

Dutka M, Bobiński R, Korbecki J. The relevance of microRNA in post-infarction left ventricular remodelling and heart failure.
Heart Fail Rev. 2019;24(4):575-86.

*Abstract**

A high-risk of morbidity and mortality is associated with myocardial infarction (MI) and postinfarction left ventricular remodeling. Because of this, current research is being carried out for learning the mechanisms of unfavorable left ventricular remodeling after an MI.

New biomarkers are also being desired that would help in early identification of patients who have a high-risk of postinfarction remodeling and dysfunction of the left ventricle. Recently, more experimental data exists that confirms the significance of microRNA in case of cardiovascular diseases. MicroRNAs have been confirmed to be stable in systemic circulation and can be measured directly in the blood of patients. It has been reported that significant changes occur in the concentrations of many types of microRNA in MI and heart failure patients. Several types of microRNA are also presently being intensively researched with respect to their usefulness as markers of cardiomyocyte necrosis, as well as predictors of the postinfarction heart failure development. In this article, a summary of the latest knowledge on the importance of microRNA in postinfarction left ventricular remodeling and heart failure is given.

"MicroRNA plays a big role in postinfarction left ventricular remodeling and heart failure. Can we manipulate it to modify or reverse heart failure especially because it involves a group of patients that have a high risk of morbidity and mortality?"

COMMENT

Cardiovascular diseases are still a principal cause of death in developed countries, in spite of significant progress in its treatment. This is mainly because of acute coronary syndromes. Recent methods used in the treatment of myocardial infarction (MI) patients have resulted in a significantly lower early mortality from this disease. However, a lot of MI patients suffer from unfavorable left ventricular remodeling and heart failure development. Heart failure still remains a very serious clinical problem, despite improvements in its treatment. It causes high mortality; many patients suffer from severe symptoms in spite of optimal treatment; because of this reason, efforts are being taken to understand the mechanisms determining unfavorable left ventricular remodeling and heart failure development among some MI patients, and to learn about the protective mechanisms that can safeguard other patients from such remodeling. MicroRNAs (miRNAs) are a group of small and non-coding RNA molecules that regulate the expression of genes at the transcriptional and post-transcriptional stages. MiRNAs are the most numerous group of small regulatory RNAs, referred to as srRNAs. The srRNAs comprise miRNAs that play a role in gene silencing at the post-transcriptional or transcriptional stage, small interfering RNAs (siRNAs), which silence genes at post-transcriptional stage, and transacting siRNAs, antisense iRNAs, and pivi-interactive RNAs. There is a growing interest in miRNAs occurring in the humans because of the role that the molecules play in several significant physiological and pathological processes. It has been reported that miRNAs in people take part in the regulation of processes such as the differentiation of skeletal muscle cells, the differentiation of hematopoietic stem cells, embryogenesis, neurogenesis, angiogenesis, differentiation of mononuclear cells, the formation and activity of immune system cells, and insulin secretion. Their significance has also been confirmed in conditions like cancer, metabolic diseases, infections, autoimmune diseases, cancer, and cardiovascular diseases. Recently, close attention has been paid particularly to some miRNAs because of their participation in the regulation of the function of the endothelial cells and vascular endothelium present in the heart, along with their effect on left ventricular remodeling following an MI. Many studies are finding proof of the key role miRNAs play in MI as well as in the occurrence of postinfarction left ventricular remodeling; because of the growing body of data that confirms the important role of several miRNAs in postinfarction heart remodeling and heart failure, miRNAs can be seen only as potential diagnostic or prognostic markers, as well as potential therapeutic targets for this group of diseases. The relationships reported so far between various types of miRNA and cardiomyocyte apoptosis processes and myocardium fibrosis have opened the way to the search for detailed pathogenic mechanisms that form the basis of these relationships. The authors brilliantly elucidate the processes involved and stimulate to continue the search for potential therapies in the field of those cardiovascular diseases, for which there is currently a severe lack of effective treatment.

(Key Message)

⊙ *In this article, authors discuss the growing body of data that confirms the important role of different miRNAs in postinfarction heart remodeling and heart failure. Based on this body of evidence, miRNAs can be seen not only as potential diagnostic or prognostic markers, but also as potential therapeutic targets for altering disease outcomes.*

ARTICLE 9

Mitochondrial Membrane Transporters and Metabolic Switch in Heart Failure

Kumar V, Kumar STR, Kartha CC. Mitochondrial membrane transporters and metabolic switch in heart failure. *Heart Fail Rev. 2019;24(2):255-67.*

*Abstract**

In the progression of cardiac failure, mitochondrial dysfunction is widely identified as one of the major factors. Key factors that regulate mitochondrial function in the normal heart include mitochondrial uptake of metabolic substrates and their utilization for ATP synthesis; electron transport chain activity; reactive oxygen species (ROS) levels; ion homeostasis; mitochondrial biogenesis; and dynamics as well as levels of ROS in the mitochondria. Alterations in any of these functions lead to adverse outcomes in heart failure. Oxidative stress and iron imbalance are also considered as major factors for the evolution of heart failure, aging-associated pathological changes in the heart, and cardiac hypertrophy. Mitochondrial ATP-binding cassette (ABC) transporters play an important role in regulation of iron metabolism and maintenance of the redox status in cells. Deficiency of mitochondrial ABC transporters is related to impairment in mitochondrial electron transport chain complex activity, iron overload, and increase in levels of ROS—all of which can lead to mitochondrial dysfunction. We aimed to discuss role of mitochondrial ABC transporters in the mitochondrial metabolism and metabolic switch; alterations in the functioning of ABC transporters in heart failure; and mitochondrial ABC transporters as possible targets for therapeutic intervention in heart failure.

---

*Redrafted abstract

"Mitochondrial dysfunction is commonly identified as a significant factor in progression of cardiac failure and contributes to adverse outcomes. Is there a way in which we can modulate their function to alter the progression and outcome in heart failure?"

COMMENT

Cardiac failure is a progressive condition in which decreased cardiac output arising from poor heart muscle contractility leads to an insufficient supply of blood to organs and therefore an impaired supply of oxygen vis-a-vis demand. Worldwide, millions of people die due to cardiac failure every year. Major drugs used for management of heart failure are vasodilators, beta-blockers, inotropic agents, and diuretics. These drugs unload the heart, reduce blood pressure, and maintain systolic/diastolic function of a compromised heart. Recent heart failure treatment strategies only help to minimize cardiac dysfunction; these do not reverse the diseased heart to a healthy condition. In patients with heart failure, mortality is 15% and rehospitalization is 35%. Mitochondrial dysfunction is widely identified as one of the major accompaniments of heart failure. Distinct features of mitochondrial dysfunction related to heart failure include alterations in mitochondrial dynamics (fusion, fission and autophagy); membrane potential and ion homeostasis; switch in substrate metabolism; and increase in ROS and other free radicals (hydroxyl and nitric oxide). In this review, the authors evaluate the mitochondrial alterations in heart failure

with focus on the role of mitochondrial membrane transporters in metabolic switch, mitochondrial dysfunction, and worsening of cardiac failure. Mitochondrial dysfunction is one of the major accompaniments of cardiac failure resulting from structural changes (disruption of one or both membranes, altered organization, and membrane composition), impaired quality control or dynamics (deteriorated mitochondrial fission and fusion as well as biogenesis, changes in membrane potential, and mitophagy processes), and functional alterations (diminished/reduced ETC complex activity and ATP production). Mitochondria in the normal heart are well organized and consists of tightly packed cristae and matrix; whereas, mitochondria in the failing heart are swollen and have decreased matrix density. This article explores the evidence to show that energy deficiency in the severely hypertrophic heart as well as in failing hearts can be corrected in many ways. Maintaining the balance between accumulation and utilization of substrates and enhancing cardiac energetics by manipulating cardiac energy metabolism is an adjunctive approach for managing heart failure patients.

Key Message

⦿ Mitochondrial dysfunction is commonly identified as a significant heart failure accompaniment. Alterations in the mitochondrial dynamics (fusion, fission and autophagy), membrane potential and ion homeostasis, switch in substrate metabolism, and increase in ROS and other free radicals (hydroxyl and nitric oxide) are distinct features of mitochondrial dysfunction related with cardiac failure. Maintaining the balance between substrate accumulation and utilization and enhancing cardiac energetics by manipulating cardiac energy metabolism is an adjunctive approach in the management of heart failure patients.

ARTICLE 10

Right Ventricular Mechanical Pattern in Health and Disease: Beyond Longitudinal Shortening

Kovács A, Lakatos B, Tokodi M, et al. Right ventricular mechanical pattern in health and disease: Beyond longitudinal shortening.
Heart Fail Rev. 2019;24(4):511-20.

*Abstract**

Right ventricular (RV) function has been proved to be a prognostic factor in cardiac failure with reduced and preserved ejection fraction as well as in pulmonary hypertension. RV function is also known to be a cornerstone in the management of new clinical issues, like grown-up congenital heart disease patients or mechanical circulatory support devices. In spite of the notable amount of circumferentially oriented myofibers in the subepicardial layer of the RV myocardium, the nonlongitudinal motion directions are usually neglected in the daily evaluation of RV function by echocardiography (ECG). However, the complex RV contraction pattern includes several motion components along three anatomically relevant axes: (1) longitudinal shortening with traction of the tricuspid annulus toward the apex, (2) radial motion of free wall often referred as the "bellows effect", and (3) anteroposterior shortening of the chamber by stretching the free wall over the septum. Advanced echocardiographic techniques, like speckle-tracking and 3D ECG, allow an in-depth characterization of RV mechanical pattern, and thus provide better understanding of RV systolic and diastolic function. In the current review, existing knowledge related to RV mechanical adaptation to the pressure- and/or volume-overloaded states as well as other physiologic/pathologic conditions are summarized.

> *"The right ventricular function is a cornerstone in the management of new clinical issues, specifically cardiac failure, mechanical circulatory support devices, and grown-up congenital heart disease. We need an in-depth understanding of the right ventricle and how it is different from the left ventricle (LV) to manage various clinical scenarios relevant in our daily practice as clinicians"*

COMMENT

In comparison to the left ventricle (LV), the anatomy and function of which have been the subjects of intensive research, right ventricular (RV) morphology and mechanics have been traditionally less studied in contemporary science. During past few decades, new diagnostic techniques and significant studies on epidemiology have brought RV function back into the scientific limelight. RV function is proved to be a prognostic factor in cardiac failure with reduced and preserved ejection fraction as well as in pulmonary hypertension. RV function is also considered to be a cornerstone in the management of novel clinical issues, e.g. grown-up congenital heart disease patients

*Redrafted abstract

or mechanical circulatory support devices. In this review, existing knowledge related to RV mechanics in different overload conditions is summarized by author and the role of nonlongitudinal contraction of the chamber and its evaluation have been emphasized. Avoiding RV failure is presently a major and important goal, e.g. in HFpEF, CHD, and pulmonary hypertension patients. For assessment and monitoring of RV morphology and function, ECG is the first-line modality. Two-dimensional approaches, however, do not provide a good estimation of the nonlongitudinal contraction of the chamber. Particularly, the subepicardial layer of the RV myocardium comprises circumferentially oriented myofibers (which play an important role in the complex contraction pattern). Nevertheless, more prospective studies are required for assessing the clinical value of in-depth characterization of RV mechanics. While it seems that pressure overload affects the RV in a uniform way, the mechanical characterization of volume-overloaded RV is more complex. Beside contractility, the preload and afterload determine RV function; effect of pericardial constraint should not be neglected. Surgical procedures cause an instant shift in functional pattern. For providing a clinical recommendation for assessment of RV function, it is significant to emphasize that the sole assessment of longitudinal shortening does not grant sufficient information related to majority of RV-related pathological conditions. If 2D ECG is applied, a detailed strategy by multiple parameters is suggested, including measures that conventionally refer to the longitudinal shortening [tricuspid annular plane systolic excursion (TAPSE) and tissue Doppler imaging] and, significantly, adding others that will at least partly include radial shortening (FAC). The incremental diagnostic and prognostic value of the speckle-tracking-derived longitudinal strain is established for evaluation of the RV as well, and should be also implemented. However, in both the clinical and research perspectives, 3D ECG-based geometric and functional RV characterization can represent a real breakthrough. By big vendors and by custom development, many software solutions enter the arena to also quantify the nonlongitudinal component of the RV mechanical pattern. Knowledge gap in our understanding of the adaptation of RV shape and function appears to be narrowing because of advanced imaging modalities. As for the LV, the next steps in RV research activity are segmental and subsequent motion pattern analyses. Armed with this information, we are in a position to treat RV failure better and improve clinical outcomes.

Key Message

⊙ *Understanding right ventricular anatomy and physiology and its differences from the left ventricle determines the overall success in the management of heart failure patients and improves clinical outcomes.*

Section 2

Heart Failure Clinics

Section Editor: Sandeep Seth

Introducing Nurse-led Heart Failure Clinics in Swedish Primary Care Settings

Liljeroos M, Strömberg A. Introducing nurse-led heart failure clinics in Swedish primary care settings. *Eur J Heart Fail. 2019;21(1):103-9.*

Abstract*

Background: Clinical guidelines recommend that patients with heart failure (HF) should receive structured multidisciplinary care at nurse-led HF clinics, so that treatment can be optimized and preventable readmissions can be avoided. Presently, about all Swedish hospitals have HF clinics with specialist-trained nurses, but there is paucity of HF clinics in primary care (PC).

Aims: In this study, there were 2-fold aims—first, to assess the effects of systematically implementing nurse-led HF clinics in PC settings with respect to evidence-based HF treatment and hospital healthcare utilization, and second, to find experience of patients of HF clinics in PC.

Methods and Results: This study had a pre-post design. Annual measurements, related to in-hospital healthcare consumption and medical treatment, were taken between 2010 and 2017. We compared data from 2011 to 2017 after implementation of HF clinics in PC in one county council Sweden with baseline data collected before implementation in 2010. There was a significant reduction in the number of HF-related hospital admissions by 27%, HF hospital days by 27.3% (p <0.001), and HF emergency room visits by 24% (p <0.001) after the implementation of HF clinics in PC. In addition, patients were medically treated as per guidelines to a higher extent; there was satisfaction among patients with the care they got at the PC HF clinic.
Conclusion: Nurse-led PC HF clinics appear to be efficient in decreasing the need for in-hospital care and providing person-centered care of high quality.

COMMENT

This is a simple elegant study showing the benefit of about 25% reduction in admissions and emergency room visits by introducing heart failure clinics in primary care.

*Redrafted abstract

ARTICLE 2

Nurse-led Heart Failure Clinics are Associated with Reduced Mortality but not Heart Failure Hospitalization

Savarese G, Lund LH, Dahlström U, et al. Nurse-led heart failure clinics are associated with reduced mortality but not heart failure hospitalization.
J Am Heart Assoc. 2019;8(10):e011737.

*Abstract**

Background: In heart failure (HF) guidelines, follow-up in a nurse-led HF clinic is recommended. However, its association with outcomes is still under controversy, as past studies have included few and highly selected patients. Therefore, large studies of "real-world" samples are required. We aimed to evaluate the independent predictors along with prognosis of planned referral to nurse-led HF clinics.

Methods and Results: In this study, data from the SwedeHF (Swedish HF Registry) was analyzed by using multivariable logistic regressions for identifying independent predictors of planned referral to a nurse-led HF clinic. Multivariable Cox regressions were used for testing associations between planned referral and outcomes (HF hospitalization, all-cause death, and their composite). A follow-up in a nurse-led HF clinic was planned for 39% of 40,992 patients.

The independent characteristics that were found to be associated with planned referral included short duration of HF, clinical markers of more severe HF, like higher New York Heart Association class, lower ejection fraction, and N-terminal pro-B-type natriuretic peptide, and low blood pressure, as well as male sex, cohabitating versus living alone, more use of HF treatments, and fewer comorbidities. Following adjustments, the planned referral to nurse-led HF clinic was observed to be associated with decreased mortality and HF hospitalization/mortality, but not HF hospitalization alone.

Conclusion: In this nationwide registry, 39% of our recognized HF cohort was planned to be referred to nurse-led HF clinic. Planned referral showed more severe HF, and also family- and sex-related factors; it was independently associated with reduced risk of death, but not of HF hospitalization.

COMMENT

This is a referred high-risk population and planned referral leads to lower mortality and higher use of medications.

*Redrafted abstract

ARTICLE 3

An Outpatient Heart Failure Clinic Reduces 30-day Readmission and Mortality Rates for Discharged Patients: Process and Preliminary Outcomes

Koser KD, Ball LS, Homa JK, et al. An outpatient heart failure clinic reduces 30-day readmission and mortality rates for discharged patients: Process and preliminary outcomes.
J Nurs Res. 2018;26(6):393-8.

Abstract*

Background: The establishment of first outpatient heart failure clinic (HFC) in Western New York was done in a large private cardiology practice with the objective of decreasing 30-day all-cause rehospitalization and inpatient mortality.

Purpose: We aimed to evaluate the process and outcomes of patients in this independent outpatient HFC. Our specific aims were—(1) to explain the outpatient care strategies used; and (2) to evaluate whether the HFC decreased 30-day all-cause rehospitalizations and inpatient mortality by comparing HFC data with census data.

Methods: In this study, a retrospective chart analysis was done on 415 adults who were included in the target HFC after hospitalization for heart failure (HF). Using frequency comparison and descriptive statistics, data were summarized. One-sample chi-square tests were performed for testing observed values in the study sample against the census data.

Results: Patients in HFC were less likely experienced a hospital readmission within 30 days of discharge (69% reduction within the study period, $p < 0.001$).
   Patients were observed acutely following discharge, received multiple medication adjustments, and telephonic follow-up was continued. There were statistically lower inpatient mortality rates in HFC (1.2% vs. 11.6% national average, $p < 0.001$), which is probably a result of the HFC care regimen and referrals to palliative care (17%).

Conclusion: The findings of this study show the significance of establishing an outpatient HFC in association with hospitals, which is aimed at decreasing the 30-day all-cause readmissions and inpatient mortality, along with referral for palliative care when indicated.

COMMENT

The design of this study is useful to structure a program for any hospital, as it covers the care from hospital admission to 60 days postdischarge. The heart failure management team covering a group of hospitals is contacted within 48 hours of admission and this team keeps eyes on the patient charts and the patient till discharge and is in touch with the patient till 60 days postdischarge. This study shows reduction in morbidity and mortality.

*Redrafted abstract

Section 3

Registries

Section Editor: Hari Krishnan

ARTICLE 1

In-hospital and Three-year Outcomes of Heart Failure Patients in South India: The Trivandrum Heart Failure Registry

Sanjay G, Jeemon P, Agarwal A, et al. In-hospital and three-year outcomes of heart failure patients in South India: The Trivandrum Heart Failure Registry.
J Card Fail. 2018;24(12):842-8.

Abstract*

Background: There is paucity of long-term data from low- and middle-income countries related to outcomes of participants hospitalized with heart failure (HF).

Methods and Results: In 2013, total 1,205 participants from 18 hospitals in Thiruvananthapuram, India were included in the Trivandrum Heart Failure Registry (THFR). Data related to patients regarding demographics, clinical presentation, treatment, and outcomes were collected. Survival analyses were performed, groups were compared, and the association between heart failure (HF) type and mortality was evaluated, by adjusting for covariates predicting mortality in a global HF risk score. The mean [standard deviation (SD)] age of participants was 61.2 (13.7) years. Ischemic heart disease was the most common cause of HF (in 72% participants). The in-hospital mortality rate was found to be higher for participants who had heart failure with reduced ejection fraction (HFrEF, 9.7%) in comparison to those with heart failure with preserved ejection fraction (HFpEF, 4.8%; p = 0.003). After 3 years, death occurred in 44.8% (n = 540) participants. The all-cause mortality rate was found to be lower for participants with HFpEF (40.8%) in comparison to HFrEF (46.2%, p = 0.049). In multivariable models, older age [hazard ratio (HR) 1.24 per decade, 95% confidence interval (CI) 1.15–1.33], New York Heart Association functional class IV symptoms (HR 2.80, 95% CI 1.43–5.48), and higher serum creatinine (HR 1.12 per mg/dL, 95% CI 1.04–1.22) were noted to be associated with all-cause mortality.

Conclusion: Participants with HF in the THFR were noted to have high 3-year all-cause mortality. Targeted hospital-based quality improvement initiatives are required for improvement in survival during and after hospitalization for HF.

*Redrafted abstract

COMMENT

There are no studies which report the long-term outcome of patients with HF from India. The Trivandrum Heart Failure Registry, the first organized hospital-based HF registry from an LMIC, reports the long-term outcome of patients with HF. The 90-day and 1-year outcomes have already been published. This article reports the 3-year outcome data. The 3-year mortality was 45%, which was very similar to HFrEF and HFpEF. The factors, which were associated with higher mortality, were lack of guideline-directed medical therapy and readmissions. The high mortality rates at 3 years highlight an important role for hospital-based quality improvement initiatives for improving clinical care for patients who have HF in India.

ARTICLE 2

Target Doses of Heart Failure Medical Therapy and Blood Pressure: Insights from the CHAMP-HF Registry

Peri-Okonny PA, Mi X, Khariton Y, et al. Target doses of heart failure medical therapy and blood pressure: Insights from the CHAMP-HF registry.
JACC Heart Fail. 2019;7(4):350-8.

*Abstract**

Background: Patients who have heart failure with reduced ejection fraction (HFrEF) are occasionally titrated to the recommended doses of guideline-directed medical therapy (GDMT). The association between systolic blood pressure (SBP) and achieving GDMT target doses is not studied properly.

Methods and Results: Patients who were enrolled in the CHAMP-HF (Change the Management of Patients with Heart Failure) Registry without documented intolerance to angiotensin receptor blockers (ARBs), angiotensin-converting enzyme (ACE) inhibitors, beta-blockers (BBs), and angiotensin receptor-neprilysin inhibitors (ARNIs) were assessed at the time of enrollment. We estimated the proportion receiving target doses {percentage of target dose [95% confidence interval (CI)]} based on the latest American College of Cardiology/American Heart Association/Heart Failure Society of America heart failure guidelines at baseline among all of the patients,

*Redrafted abstract

and by SBP category (≥110 vs. <110 mm Hg). Out of 3,095 patients who were eligible for analysis, 78.2% (n = 2,421) had SBP 110 mm Hg or more.

The proportion of patients who received target doses were 18.7% (95% CI 17.3–20.0%; BB), 10.8% (95% CI 9.7–11.9%; ARB/ACE inhibitor), and 2.0% (95% CI 1.5–2.5%; ARNI). In patients with SBP less than 110 mm Hg (n = 674), 17.5% (95% CI 14.6–20.4%; BB), 6.2% (95% CI 4.4–8.1%; ARB/ACE inhibitor), and 1.8% (95% CI 0.8–2.8%; ARNI) were receiving target doses. In patients with SBP 110 mm Hg or more (n = 2,421), 19.0% (95% CI 17.4–20.6%; BB), 12.1% (95% CI 10.8–13.4%; ARB/ACE inhibitor), and 2.0% (95% CI 1.5–2.6%; ARNI) were receiving target doses.

Conclusion: In a large, contemporary registry of outpatients who had chronic HFrEF and were eligible for treatment with BBs and ARNI/ARB/ACE inhibitor, less than 20% of patients were receiving target doses, even among those with SBP 110 mm Hg or more.

COMMENT

The intake of evidence-based therapies is abysmally low in patients with heart failure (HF). Among those receiving evidence-based therapies, only a small percentage of patients are receiving the target doses. These two studies from the Change the Management of Patients with Heart Failure (CHAMP-HF) again show the same results. In this study, most of the patients were receiving target doses of mineralocorticoid receptor antagonist (MRA) therapy (77%), while number of patients receiving target doses of ARB/ACE inhibitor were 17%, ARNI (14%), and beta-blockers (28%). In patients who were eligible for all of the classes of medication, only 1% were receiving target doses of ARNI/ARB/ACE inhibitor, beta-blocker, and MRA simultaneously.

The second study which assessed the BP levels and titration to target doses registry shows that less than 20% of patients with HF receive the target doses. The reason most cited for not titrating to target doses is the fear of hypotension. However, this study shows that even in patients with SBP >110 mm Hg, less than 20% of patients receive target doses. The Indian scenario is not much different. The Trivandrum Heart Failure Registry shows that only 25% of the patients even receive the drugs; the data on how many receive the target doses are not available. Another sub-study of CHAMP-HF has shown that most eligible HFrEF patients did not receive target doses of medical therapy at any point during follow-up, as there were no significant alterations during drug therapy on follow-up, and few patients had doses which increased over time. This points to the need for Quality Improvement Programs aimed at physicians and healthcare workers and improvement in practice patterns.

ARTICLE 3

Medical Therapy for Heart Failure with Reduced Ejection Fraction: The CHAMP-HF Registry

Greene SJ, Butler J, Albert NM, et al. Medical therapy for heart failure with reduced ejection fraction: The CHAMP-HF registry.
J Am Coll Cardiol. 2018;72(4):351-66.

*Abstract**

Background: It is strongly recommended by the guidelines that patients who have heart failure with reduced ejection fraction (HFrEF) should be treated with various medications that are proven to improve clinical outcomes, as tolerated. In contemporary outpatient, degree to which gaps in medication use and dosing persist is still not clear.

Methods and Results: The CHAMP-HF (Change the Management of Patients with Heart Failure) Registry enrolled outpatients in the United States. Inclusion criteria included those outpatients who had chronic HFrEF and were receiving at least one oral medication for the management of heart failure (HF). Patients were characterized by baseline use and the dose of angiotensin II receptor blocker (ARB)/angiotensin-converting enzyme (ACE) inhibitor, angiotensin receptor-neprilysin inhibitor (ARNI), mineralocorticoid receptor antagonist (MRA), and beta-blocker. Patient-level factors that were associated with use of medication were examined.

Total 3,518 patients from 150 cardiology practices and primary care were included. The mean age of the patients was 66 ± 13 years; out of these, 29% were female; and mean ejection fraction (EF) was 29 ± 8%. The number of patients who were not prescribed ARB/ARNI/ACE inhibitor was 27%; beta-blocker was not prescribed in 33%, and MRA therapy was not prescribed to 67% patients. At the time when medications were prescribed, majority of the patients were receiving target doses of MRA therapy (77%); whereas, 28% patients were receiving target doses of beta-blocker, 17% (ARB/ACE inhibitor), and 14% (ARNI). In patients who were eligible for all classes of medication, only 1% patients were receiving target doses of ARB/ARNI/ACE inhibitor, beta-blocker, and MRA simultaneously. In adjusted models, old age, more severe functional class, lower blood pressure, renal insufficiency, and recent HF hospitalization usually supported less utilization of medication or dose. Social and economic characteristics were not found to be independently associated with use or dose of medication.

Conclusion: In this contemporary outpatient HFrEF registry, there were significant gaps in utilization and dosing of guideline-directed medical therapy. Many clinical factors were found to be associated with use of medication and dosage prescribed. There is an urgent need of strategies for improving guideline-directed use of HFrEF medications; these findings may inform targeted approaches to optimize the outpatient medical treatment.

*Redrafted abstract

COMMENT

The intake of evidence-based therapies is abysmally low in patients with heart failure (HF). Among those receiving evidence-based therapies, only a small percentage of patients are receiving the target doses. These two studies from the Change the Management of Patients with Heart Failure (CHAMP-HF) again show the same results. In this study, most of the patients were receiving target doses of mineralocorticoid receptor antagonist (MRA) therapy (77%), while number of patients receiving target doses of ARB/ACE inhibitor were 17%, ARNI (14%), and beta-blockers (28%). In patients who were eligible for all of the classes of medication, only 1% were receiving target doses of ARNI/ARB/ACE inhibitor, beta-blocker, and MRA simultaneously.

The second study which assessed the BP levels and titration to target doses registry shows that less than 20% of patients with HF receive the target doses. The reason most cited for not titrating to target doses is the fear of hypotension. However, this study shows that even in patients with SBP >110 mm Hg, less than 20% of patients receive target doses. The Indian scenario is not much different. The Trivandrum Heart Failure Registry shows that only 25% of the patients even receive the drugs; the data on how many receive the target doses are not available. Another sub-study of CHAMP-HF has shown that most eligible HFrEF patients did not receive target doses of medical therapy at any point during follow-up, as there were no significant alterations during drug therapy on follow-up, and few patients had doses which increased over time. This points to the need for Quality Improvement Programs aimed at physicians and healthcare workers and improvement in practice patterns.

Note: As per author's instruction Comment-text for Articles 2 and 3 will be same.

ARTICLE 4

Prevalence, Risk Factors, and Significance of Iron Deficiency and Anemia in Nonischemic Heart Failure Patients with Reduced Ejection Fraction from a Himachal Pradesh Heart Failure Registry

Negi PC, Dev M, Paul P, et al. Prevalence, risk factors, and significance of iron deficiency and anemia in nonischemic heart failure patients with reduced ejection fraction from a Himachal Pradesh heart failure registry. *Indian Heart J. 2018;70 Suppl 3:S182-8.*

Abstract*

Background: This study was aimed at estimating the prevalence, risk determinants, and clinical significance of iron deficiency and anemia among patients having nonischemic heart failure (HF) with reduced ejection fraction (HFrEF).

Methods and Results: In a prospective tertiary care hospital-based heart failure registry, 226 consecutive patients with HFrEF diagnosed on the basis of left ventricular ejection fraction ≤45% and absence of coronary artery luminal narrowing of >50% were included. Hemoglobin (Hb), serum ferritin, and transferrin saturation levels were measured in all patients. Patients who had New York Heart Association functional class III/IV were classified as patients with advanced HF. Multivariable logistic regression modeling was done for assessing risk determinants of the iron deficiency and anemia as well as their clinical significance as the risk factors for advanced HF. Odds ratio (OR) with 95% confidence interval (CI) was reported as estimates of strength of association between the exposure and the outcome variables. Iron deficiency was prevalent in 58.8% (52.2–65.1%) and anemia in 35.8% (29.8–42.3%) of patients.

Female gender [OR 3.5 (95% CI 1.9–6.5)]; vegetarian diet [OR 2.5 (95% CI 1.4–4.6)]; and history of bleeding [OR 11.7 (95% CI 1.4–101.2)] were found to be significantly associated with iron deficiency. Diabetes [OR 3.0 (95% CI 1.40–6.5)]; history of bleeding [OR 13.0 (95% CI 2.3–70.9)]; estimated glomerular filtration rate [OR 0.98 (95% CI 0.97–0.99)]; and female gender [OR 2.9 (95% CI 1.5–5.7)] showed significant association with anemia. Hb level [OR 0.82 (95% CI 0.70–0.96)] and transferrin saturation [OR 0.98 (95% CI 0.96–0.99)] showed significant inverse association with symptoms of advanced HF.

Conclusion: The common comorbidities associated with HFrEF are iron deficiency and anemia. There is a significant association of low Hb and transferrin saturation with advanced HF. These findings have significant implications in the management of HF.

COMMENT

Iron deficiency is a very significant remediable comorbidity in patients with heart failure (HF). Many reports from the western world find that the prevalence of iron deficiency is in the tune of 50% of ambulatory HF patients. This Indian study from the hilly state, Himachal Pradesh, shows that iron deficiency is very common in about two-thirds of the patients. This study reports that hemoglobin levels are not enough to diagnose iron deficiency (59% vs. 36%). Iron deficiency is associated with reduced exercise tolerance and reduced quality of life as reported in this study. To diagnose iron deficiency, we need to know the iron levels in the body. The criteria proposed by ESC for the diagnosis of iron deficiency in heart failure are serum ferritin, <100 µg/L, or ferritin, 100–300 µg/L, with transferrin saturation of <20%. The efficacy of oral iron products has not been so good, but the ESC recommendations are to use intravenous iron products, especially ferric carboxymaltose. Data from meta-analyses suggest that correcting iron deficiency reduces rehospitalization rates for heart failure and reduction in cardiovascular mortality rates.

*Redrafted abstract

ARTICLE 5

Association between Process Performance Measures and 1-year Mortality among Patients with Incident Heart Failure: A Danish Nationwide Study

Nakano A, Vinter N, Egstrup K, et al. Association between process performance measures and 1-year mortality among patients with incident heart failure: A Danish nationwide study.
Eur Heart J Qual Care Clin Outcomes. 2019;5(1):28-34.

*Abstract**

Aims: To analyze the relation between fulfillment of the performance measures supported by the clinical guidelines recommendations and 1-year mortality in incident heart failure (HF) patients in Denmark.

Methods and Results: This was a nationwide population-based follow-up study based on Danish hospital departments. Study included all of the Danish hospital departments who care for HF patients. Total 24,308 in- and outpatients diagnosed with HF in period from 2003 to 2010 were identified.

Quality of care was described as receiving the guideline-recommended processes of care: New York Heart Association classification, use of echocardiography, treatment with beta-blockers, angiotensin-converting enzyme inhibitors/angiotensin II receptor blocker, and patient education and physical training. One-year mortality was the main outcome measure. Multiple imputation and multivariable Cox proportional hazard regression were used for computing hazard ratios (HRs) for 1-year mortality adjusted for potential confounding factors. Within 1-year, 17.1% deaths were reported and the adjusted HRs ranged from 0.99 (95% CI 0.90–1.10) for beta-blocker therapy to 0.61 [95% confidence interval (CI) 0.55–0.67] for patient. It appeared that the association between meeting more performance measures and 1-year mortality follows a dose-response pattern: by using 0–25% of fulfilled measures as reference, patients fulfilling 76–100% of the performance measures with an adjusted HR of 0.43 (95% CI 0.38–0.48), while the adjusted HR was 0.96 (95% CI 0.86–1.07) for patients fulfilling between 26% and 50% of the performance measures.

Conclusion: Meeting process performance measures that reflect care in accordance with the clinical guideline recommendations was found to be correlated with substantially reduced 1-year mortality in incident HF patients.

COMMENT

This study can be read in the light of the previous paper by Per-Okoony et al. Performance measures—like protocol-based evaluation, ensuring guideline-directed therapy, planned follow-up care, ensuring drug compliance, rehabilitation including

*Redrafted abstract

an exercise program—will improve patient outcomes with HF. This large Danish study of 24,308 patients underlines this fact. For this to happen, we have to have periodic audits about our performance and corrective actions are to be taken. In a country like India, it will be very difficult to ensure the fulfillment of many of the above said measures, but the need of the hour is to improve outcomes. The simpler way of doing this is to have provider-targeted QI initiatives. Training physicians and HF nurses is one effective way.

ARTICLE 6

Machine Learning Methods Improve Prognostication, Identify Clinically Distinct Phenotypes, and Detect Heterogeneity in Response to Therapy in a Large Cohort of Heart Failure Patients

Ahmad T, Lund LH, Rao P, et al. Machine learning methods improve prognostication, identify clinically distinct phenotypes, and detect heterogeneity in response to therapy in a large cohort of heart failure patients. *J Am Heart Assoc. 2018;7(8):pii: e008081.*

Abstract*

Background: While heart failure (HF) is a complex clinical syndrome, it has been treated as a singular disease by conventional approaches to its management, resulting in insufficient care of patient and inefficient clinical trials. Hypothesis for this study was that application of advanced analytics to a large cohort of patients with HF would identify distinct patient phenotypes, enhance prognostication of outcomes, and detect heterogeneity in treatment response.

Methods and Results: The Swedish Heart Failure Registry is a national registry that collects comprehensive demographic, clinical, laboratory, and medication data and is linked to the databases having outcome information. Random forest modeling was applied for identifying predictors of 1-year survival. Cluster analysis was done and serial bootstrapping was used for its validation. Cox proportional-hazards modeling was used to assess association between clusters and survival; interaction testing was done for assessing heterogeneity in response to the HF pharmacotherapy across propensity-matched clusters.

Total 44,886 HF patients, who were enrolled in the Swedish Heart Failure Registry from 2000 to 2012, were included in the study. Excellent calibration and discrimination for survival was showed by random forest modeling (C-statistic = 0.83); whereas, left ventricular ejection fraction (LVEF) did not (C-statistic = 0.52): no meaningful differences per strata of LVEF were present (1-year survival: 80%, 81%, 83% and 84%). Cluster analysis done by using the eight highest predictive

*Redrafted abstract

variables recognized four clinically relevant subgroups of HF with marked differences in 1-year survival. Significant interactions were noted between the propensity-matched clusters (across age, sex, and LVEF and following medications: beta-blockers, angiotensin-converting enzyme inhibitors, diuretics, and nitrates, p <0.001, all).

Conclusion: In a large dataset of HF patients, machine learning algorithms accurately predicted outcomes. Cluster analysis recognized four distinct phenotypes that differed significantly in terms of outcomes and therapeutic responses. The use of these new analytical methods has the ability to improve the efficacy of present therapies and to transform future HF clinical trials.

COMMENT

Machine learning (ML) is defined by experts as an application of artificial intelligence (AI), which provides systems the ability of automatically learning and improving from experience without being explicitly programmed. Machine learning focuses on the developing computer programs that can access data and use it to learn for themselves. ML is widely believed to be able to learn complex hidden interactions from the data and has the potential to improve prognostication of outcomes, identify distinct patient phenotypes, and detect heterogeneity in treatment response, predict events such as readmission and mortality. This study evaluated the usefulness of machine learning algorithms and identified four distinct phenotypes that differed significantly in outcomes and response to therapeutics. For example, if we can identify the high-risk patient who is prone to heart failure readmissions, we can improve performance measures and try to prevent readmissions and, in turn, reduce the mortality. Such novel approaches can transform healthcare and can be utilized in resource-constrained economies like India.

ARTICLE 7

Incidence of Hospital-acquired Hyponatremia by the Dose and Type of Diuretics among Patients with Acute Heart Failure and its Association with Long-term Outcomes

Yamazoe M, Mizuno A, Kohsaka S, et al. Incidence of hospital-acquired hyponatremia by the dose and type of diuretics among patients with acute heart failure and its association with long-term outcomes.
J Cardiol. 2018;71(6):550-6.

Abstract*

Background: Although diuretics are considered to be a cornerstone therapy for acute heart failure (AHF), it can result in several disturbances in electrolyte and inversely affect the outcomes in patients.

Aims: To assess whether (1) the dose of loop diuretics during AHF treatment can predict hospital-acquired hyponatremia (HAH), (2) adding thiazide diuretics could have an impact on the development of HAH, and (3) evaluate their effect on long-term outcomes.

Methods and Results: In this study, the subjects enrolled in the multicenter AHF registry (WET-HF) were analyzed. Risk of HAH was defined as hyponatremia at time of discharge with normonatremia upon admission. It was assessed on the basis of oral nonpotassium-sparing diuretics through multivariate logistic regression analysis. In addition, one-to-one matched analysis was done on the basis of propensity scores for use of thiazide diuretics; long-term mortality was also compared.

Out of total 1,163 patients, 7.9% (n = 92) had HAH. Mean age of the patients was 72.6 ± 13.6 years; male were 62.6% of the total patients. In comparison with low-dose loop diuretics users (<40 mg, without thiazide diuretics), risk of developing HAH was significantly more among patients with thiazide diuretics, irrespective of the dose of loop diuretics (OR 2.67, 95% CI 1.13–6.34 and OR 2.31, 95% CI 1.50–5.13 for low-dose and high-dose loop diuretics, respectively). In patients without thiazide diuretics, the association was less apparent (OR 1.29, 95% CI 0.73–2.27 for high-dose loop diuretics alone). In 206 matched patients, all-cause mortality rate and cardiac mortality rate were 27% and 14% in the nonthiazide diuretics users and 50% and 30% among thiazide diuretics users, respectively (HR 2.46, 95% CI 1.29–4.69, p = 0.006 and HR 2.50, 95% CI 1.10–5.67, p = 0.028, respectively) during a follow-up of mean 19.3 months.

Conclusion: Use of thiazide diuretics, rather than loop diuretics dose, was noted to be independently associated with HAH; mortality was observed to be higher in thiazide diuretics users, even after statistical matching.

COMMENT

Hyponatremia is a very common problem among patients on diuretic therapy. Since diuretics are the cornerstone of therapy in acute decompensated heart failure (ADHF), almost all patients must be exposed to diuretics. Mild hyponatremia is defined as a serum sodium concentration between 130 mEq/L and 135 mEq/L, moderate hyponatremia as sodium concentration between 125 mEq/L and 129 mEq/L, and severe hyponatremia as serum sodium of 125 mEq/L or less. Hyponatremia is the most common electrolyte abnormality encountered in patients hospitalized with ADHF. Hyponatremia is associated with increased mortality and morbidity in patients with HF. The two common classes of diuretics in use are thiazides and loop diuretics. It was reported in reviews that 73% of cases of drug-induced hyponatremia were caused by thiazides alone while 20% by thiazide–potassium-sparing diuretics, and the loop diuretic furosemide was associated with only 7% of cases. Thiazide diuretics induce

*Redrafted abstract

hyponatremia as these drugs act exclusively in distal tubules and do not interfere with urinary concentration and the ability of arginine vasopressin in promoting the ability of arginine vasopressin. Compared to thiazides, loop diuretics do not usually cause hyponatremia as they impair both renal concentrating and diluting mechanisms.

This study also confirms the same, thiazide diuretics caused more hyponatremia than even high-dose loop diuretics. Vasopressin receptor antagonists or Vaptans have very unique features, which will help patients with HF and hyponatremia, and are increasingly utilized in the treatment of this electrolyte abnormality associated with HF.

ARTICLE 8

Early Ambulation among Hospitalized Heart Failure Patients is Associated with Reduced Length of Stay and 30-day Readmissions

Fleming LM, Zhao X, DeVore AD, et al. Early ambulation among hospitalized heart failure patients is associated with reduced length of stay and 30-day readmissions.
Circ Heart Fail. 2018;11(4):e004634.

*Abstract**

Background: In mechanically ventilated and stroke patients, early ambulation (EA) is related with improved outcomes. It is still not known whether similar association exists for patients hospitalized with acute heart failure. We aimed to evaluate whether EA in patients hospitalized with heart failure is associated with length of hospital stay, discharge disposition, 30-day postdischarge readmissions, and mortality.

Methods and Results: In this study, 369 hospitals and 285,653 heart failure patients enrolled in the Get with The Guidelines-Heart Failure Registry were included. Multivariate logistic regression with generalized estimating equations was used at the hospital level for identifying predictors of EA and for assessing the association between EA and outcomes. Total 65% patients were ambulated by day two of the hospital admission. Patient-level predictors of EA consisted of young age, male gender, and hospitalization outside of the Northeast (p <0.01, for all). Academic status and hospital size were not predictive. It was demonstrated by hospital-level analysis that those hospitals having EA rates in the top 25% were less likely to be related with a long length of stay (defined as more than 4 days) in comparison to those in the bottom 25% [odds ratio 0.83, confidence interval 0.73–0.94, p = 0.004). In a subgroup of fee-for-service Medicare beneficiaries, it was observed that hospitals in the highest quartile of rates of EA revealed statistically significant

*Redrafted abstract

24% lower 30-day readmission rates (p <0.0001). Both end-points revealed a dose-response association and statistically significant p for trend test.

Conclusion: Multivariable-adjusted hospital-level analysis reveals an association of EA with both short length of hospital stays and lower 30-day readmissions. More future prospective studies are required for validating these findings.

COMMENT

Patients admitted with acute decompensated heart failure (ADHF) are being advised to have graded careful ambulation. In this large study from the Get with Guidelines Study (369 hospitals and 285,653 patients), those who had early ambulation (<2 days) were compared to those who had ambulation later. About 65% of the patients had early ambulation. Multivariable-adjusted hospital-level analysis reveals an association of EA with both short length of hospital stays and lower 30-days readmissions. Early ambulation is an inexpensive intervention, which can be considered as a process measure or as an additional quality metric to evaluate the care of patients hospitalized with ADHF. We know that 2% of the healthcare budget is channeled toward the management of HF, mostly in in-patients. It burdens the healthcare system and necessitates multiple readmissions and longer lengths of stay. If proven in randomized trials, low-cost interventions like early ambulation may help to improve their outcomes.

ARTICLE 9

Incidence, Predictors, and Outcome Associations of Dyskalemia in Heart Failure with Preserved, Mid-range, and Reduced Ejection Fraction

Savarese G, Xu H, Trevisan M, et al. Incidence, predictors, and outcome associations of dyskalemia in heart failure with preserved, mid-range, and reduced ejection fraction.
ACC Heart Fail. 2019;7(1):65-76.

*Abstract**

Background: Dyskalemia (dysK) in real-world heart failure (HF) is not sufficiently characterized. Fear of dysK may result in less use or overdosing of renin–angiotensin–aldosterone system (RAAS) inhibitors.

**Redrafted abstract

Methods and Results: In this analysis, patients, who were enrolled in the SwedeHF (Swedish Heart Failure) Registry between 2006 and 2011 in Stockholm, Sweden, were included. By multivariate Cox regression analysis, independent predictors of dysK within 1-year were identified. By time-dependent Cox models, the outcomes associated with the incident dysK [all-cause death, HF, and other cardiovascular disease (CVD) hospitalizations] within 1-year from baseline were evaluated. Out of total 5,848 patients included in study, 24.4% had hyperkalemia [hyperK (K >5.0 mmol/L)] at least once, and 10.2% experienced moderate/severe hyperK (K >5.5 mmol/L). Adjusted risk of moderate or severe hyperK was highest in heart failure with preserved ejection fraction (HFpEF) and heart failure with mid-range ejection fraction (HFmrEF). Similar to this, 20.3% patients experienced minimum one episode of hypokalemia [hypoK (K <3.5 mmol/L)], and 3.7% experienced severe hypoK (K <3.0 mmol/L). Adjusted risk of any hypoK was observed to be highest in HFpEF. Following were the independent predictors of both hypoK and hyperK: gender; baseline potassium and estimated glomerular filtration rate (eGFR); low hemoglobin; higher New York Heart Association functional class; chronic obstructive pulmonary disease (COPD); and inpatient status. Incident dysK was observed to be associated with increased risk of mortality. Moreover, hypoK was related to increase in CVD hospitalizations (HF-related excluded). No association was found between dysK and HF hospitalization risk, irrespective of EF.

Conclusion: Dyskalemia is common finding in HF and is related with increase in mortality. Risk of moderate/severe hyperK was found to be highest in HFpEF and HFmrEF; risk of hypoK was noted to be highest in HFpEF. Relevant predictors of dysK occurrence were low hemoglobin, HF severity, baseline high and low potassium, low eGFR, and COPD.

COMMENT

Both hyperkalemia and hypokalemia are common accompaniments of heart failure (HF) therapy. This is related to the hemodynamic consequences of HF leading to altered fluid dynamics, associated renal impairment and due to pharmacotherapy, which includes diuretics and drugs acting on the RAAS system. In this real-world cohort of 5,848 patients from the Swedish HF registry, both hyponatremia and hyperkalemia were reported and were associated with higher mortality. Hyperkalemia was reported in 24% of patients and hypokalemia was present in 20% of patients. Interestingly, dyskalemia was more common in patients with HFpEF than in patients with HFrEF. Predictors of dysK occurrence included low hemoglobin, HF severity, high and low potassium levels at baseline, low eGFR, and COPD. Beta-blockers were noted to be associated with a lower risk of hypoK that is consistent with their role in promoting potassium shift out of cells by inhibition of sodium–potassium ATPase. Fear of dyskalemia among these patients can result into underuse or underdosing of RAAS inhibitors. The risk predictors can be used for initiating essential drugs in HF.

ARTICLE 10

Beta-blockers and 1-year Postdischarge Mortality for Heart Failure and Reduced Ejection Fraction and Slow Discharge Heart Rate

Park JJ, Park HA, Cho HJ, et al. β-blockers and 1-year postdischarge mortality for heart failure and reduced ejection fraction and slow discharge heart rate.
J Am Heart Assoc. 2019;8(4):e011121.

*Abstract**

Background: Several hospitalized patients having heart failure and reduced ejection fraction (HFrEF) have a slow heart rate at the time of discharge, and the effect of beta-blockers may be decreased among those patients. This study aimed at evaluating the variable effect of beta-blockers on clinical outcomes as per the discharge heart rate of hospitalized HFrEF patients.

Methods and Results: Total 5,625 patients hospitalized for acute heart failure (HF) were consecutively enrolled in the KorAHF (Korean Acute Heart Failure) Registry. Patients with HFrEF (left ventricular ejection fraction ≤ 40%) were included in this analysis. Slow heart rate was defined as less than 70 bpm irrespective of the use of beta-blockers. The primary outcome considered in study was 1-year all-cause postdischarge death as per the heart rate. Out of 2,932 patients with HFrEF, 29% (n = 840) had slow heart rate and 56% received beta-blockers at time of discharge. Patients having slow heart rates were old in age and with reduced 1-year mortality as compared to those with high heart rates (p <0.001). A significant interaction was noted between discharge heart rate and use of beta-blocker (p <0.001 for interaction).

When stratified, only those patients without beta-blocker prescription and having high heart rate demonstrated higher 1-year mortality. On Cox-proportional hazards regression analysis, beta-blocker prescription at discharge was found to be associated with 24% reduced risk for 1-year mortality among patients having high heart rates [hazard ratio (HR) 0.76; 95% confidence interval (CI) 0.61–0.95] but not in those having slow heart rates (HR 1.02; 95% CI 0.68–1.55).

Conclusion: Several patients with acute HF have slow discharge heart rates, and beta-blockers may have a limited effect on the HFrEF and slow discharge heart rate.

COMMENT

The heightened sympathetic activity has shown to be one of the pathogenetic mechanisms in HF. Sympathetic blockade using beta-blockers has been one of the cornerstones of treatment of HFrEF and has shown significant mortality reduction in

*Redrafted abstract

trials. One of the mechanisms by which beta-blockers produce benefit in HF is due to the reduction in heart rate.

Early initiation of beta-blockers, especially at discharge after acute heart failure, is beneficial and is recommended. The magnitude of the heart rate reduction by beta-blockers depends on the baseline heart rate. In this study from the KorAHF (Korean Acute Heart Failure) Registry, they found that beta-blocker therapy was associated with a reduced mortality risk at 1-year in patients with high heart rate but not in those with slower heart rate. This may suggest a differential effect of beta-blockers by heart rate. However, beta-blocker therapy showed a favorable effect on hospitalization for heart failure regardless of heart rate. So, this study suggests that probably not all patients benefit equally from beta-blocker therapy. Those who have a higher discharge heart rate (>70 bpm) may benefit, others may not. Since there was a benefit on rehospitalization, despite the HR, the current practice of initiating beta-blockers should continue, but risk–benefit should be assessed.

Section 4

Biomarkers

Section Editor: Uday Jadhav

ARTICLE 1

Cardiac Biomarkers in the Emergency Department: The Role of Soluble ST2 (sST2) in Acute Heart Failure and Acute Coronary Syndrome—There is Meat on the Bone

Aleksova A, Paldino A, Beltrami AP, et al. Cardiac biomarkers in the emergency department: The role of soluble ST2 (sST2) in acute heart failure and acute coronary syndrome—There is meat on the bone.
J Clin Med. 2019;8(2):270.

*Abstract**

In the field of acute cardiovascular diseases, soluble suppression of tumorigenicity 2 (sST2) has recently emerged as a promising biomarker. Many clinical studies have shown significant link between sST2 values and outcome of patients. Moreover, higher levels of sST2 are found to be associated with an increase in risk of adverse left ventricular remodeling. Thus, sST2 can represent as a beneficial tool, which can help in the risk stratification along with diagnostic and therapeutic work-up of patients in an emergency department. With this review, which was based on recent literature, sST2-assisted flowcharts were built that were applicable to three very common clinical scenarios of emergency department—type 1 and type 2 acute myocardial infarction, and acute heart failure. Specifically, sST2 levels were combined with clinical and instrumental evaluation so that to offer a practical tool for emergency medicine physicians.

COMMENT

The soluble variant of suppression of tumorigenicity 2 (ST2) leads to being overexpressed in particular pathologic conditions of the myocardial stress or injury and it is associated with immune response and inflammation.

American AHA/ACC guidelines for the management of heart failure (HF) recommend (class IIb, Level of Evidence B) that for a more appropriate risk stratification, measurement of soluble suppression of

*Redrafted abstract

tumorigenicity 2 (sST2) should be done in patients with acute decompensated heart failure (ADHF).

In contrast to the natriuretic peptides (NPs), sST2 is not influenced by either body mass index, age, renal function, or etiology of HF with lowest intraindividual variation and smallest relative change value.

The review has excellent algorithm flowcharts on ST2 in context with ADHF, type 1 myocardial infarction (MI) and type 2 MI. Summary of these algorithms are highlighted here.

For distinguishing emergency department (ED) patients with a very high-risk of ADHF, a level of 70 ng/mL constitutes a potential cutoff value. The sST2 values above about 70 ng/mL have been found to be associated with higher risk of death on short-term (30 days) and long-term (1 year) follow-up.

In patients with dyspnea and elevated NPs, sST2 levels can help to identify three classes of patients. If sST2 is less than 35 ng/mL, the diagnosis of ADHF is unusual. Among patients having 35 ≤ sST2 ≤70 ng/mL, ADHF is more common but mild-to-moderate. If sST2 is more than 70 ng/mL, ADHF is fairly common, which needs antiremodeling therapies and hospitalization.

The sST2 adds nothing to the initial diagnosis of acute myocardial infarction (AMI), its prognostic role has become noteworthy. Early levels of sST2 in AMI reflect the extent of myocardial necrosis with negative correlation with left ventricular (LV) ejection fraction at 1 day after AMI.

Early levels of sST2 have been correlated with mortality as well as with the development of new/worsening of congestive HF by 30 days after ST elevation myocardial infarction (STEMI). In majority of these patients, the peak values of sST2 occurred at 12 hours. In contrast to NT-proBNP that increases exponentially in 4 days after STEMI, the sST2 12-hour peak is followed by a significant reduction.

In patients with type 1 AMI, sST2 levels can help to identify three classes of patients. If sST2 <35 ng/mL, adverse remodeling is unlikely. In patients with 35 ≤ sST2 ≤70 ng/mL, adverse remodeling is more likely, and patients could benefit from antifibrotic therapies. If sST2 is more than 70 ng/mL, adverse remodeling is fairly common, which needs aggressive antiremodeling therapies.

In patients with type 2 AMI and elevated troponin levels, sST2 levels can help to identify three classes of patients. If sST2 <35 ng/mL, adverse remodeling is unlikely. In patients having 35 ≤ sST2 ≤70 ng/mL, adverse remodeling is more common, and patients can get benefit from antifibrotic therapies. If sST2 is more than 70 ng/mL, a significant activation of fibrotic and neurohormonal pathways is likely.

ARTICLE 2

Soluble ST2—A New Biomarker in Heart Failure

Patric B, Camille A, Mauro I, et al. Soluble ST2—A new biomarker in heart failure. *Cardiovasc Med. 2019;22:w02008.*

*Abstract**

There is an essential role of cardiovascular biomarkers in the diagnosis, risk stratification, and treatment of patients having cardiac diseases and especially heart failure patients. However, confounding comorbidities limit the accuracy of most of the biomarkers, which renders their interpretation to be difficult. It is said that relatively new biomarker soluble suppression of tumorigenicity 2 (sST2) reflects myocardial wall stress and fibrosis pathway activation and is less dependent on common confounders. Elevated levels of sST2 predict both rehospitalization and mortality in patients with acute heart failure. Patients with chronic heart failure with levels of sST2 responsive to medical treatment have better outcome. However, elevation in levels of sST2 in the absence of heart disease or heart failure is not uncommon and limits its use for diagnosis in a general nonheart failure population. This review represents the participants' presentations and discussions at the Swiss Working Group's first meeting on cardiovascular biomarkers in Zurich, Switzerland, in September 2018.

It also shows present Swiss experience with sST2 and shows areas of uncertainty, specifically the requirement of identifying the exact pathway of sST2 in cardiac disease and specifies its clinical implications for subgroups of nonheart failure and heart failure patients.

COMMENT

Heart failure (HF) patients presenting with dyspnea are accurately diagnosed by B-type natriuretic peptide (BNP); it also predicts future events when a cutoff level of 100 ng/mL is used. Cutoff level of 300 pg/mL for N-terminal pro-B-type natriuretic peptide (NT-proBNP) has been proposed with a 98% predictive value to exclude acute HF.

Age-independent clinical conditions that lead to increase in inflammation, wall stress, and macrophage activation raise soluble suppression of tumorigenicity 2 (sST2) levels and thus result in increase in cardiac fibrosis. The sST2 is expressed by other organs also and is increased in several liver diseases and increase in sST2 levels is not specific for cardiac failure.

For males, mean normal values of sST2 are 24.9 ng/mL (95% nonparametric reference interval 8.6–49.3 ng/mL) and for females are 16.9 ng/mL (95% nonparametric reference interval 7.2–33.5 ng/mL). Recent cutoff level that indicates good outcome in ambulatory patients of HF is 35 ng/mL. In the absence of HF, 10–18% of men and 2–8% of women will have values more than this cutoff level.

It remains to be seen whether use of ST2 as single biomarker in HF will supersede the use of multiple biomarkers for predicting death, cardiovascular events and HF.

*Redrafted abstract

ARTICLE 3

Cardiovascular Biomarkers in Patients with Acute Decompensated Heart Failure Randomized to Sacubitril-valsartan or Enalapril in the PIONEER-HF Trial

Morrow DA, Velazquez EJ, DeVore AD, et al. Cardiovascular biomarkers in patients with acute decompensated heart failure randomized to sacubitril-valsartan or enalapril in the PIONEER-HF trial.
Eur Heart J. 2019. pii: ehz240.

*Abstract**

Aims: In patients with heart failure (HF), circulating high-sensitivity cardiac troponin (hsTn) and the soluble suppression of tumorigenicity 2 (sST2) reflect myocardial stress. Cyclic guanosine 3'5' monophosphate (cGMP) production in response to activation of natriuretic peptide receptors decreases cardiac preload and afterload. Effects of sacubitril/valsartan on these biomarkers among patients with reduced ejection fraction and acute decompensated heart failure (ADHF) were assessed.

Methods and Results: PIONEER-HF was a randomized, double-blind trial of sacubitril/valsartan versus enalapril in hospitalized patients who had ADHF following hemodynamic stabilization. Circulating hsTnT, sST2, and urinary cGMP were measured at baseline, 1, 2 (sST2, cGMP), 4, and 8 weeks (n = 694 with all baseline biomarkers). Geometric mean ratios (timepoint/baseline) were determined and compared as a sacubitril/valsartan versus enalapril ratio. In comparison to enalapril, sacubitril/valsartan resulted in a significantly greater decline in hsTnT and sST2. This effect appeared for sST2 as soon as 1 week and was significant for both at 4 weeks with a 16% greater reduction in hsTnT ($p < 0.001$) and a 9% greater reduction in sST2 ($p = 0.0033$). Serial urinary cGMP significantly increased with sacubitril/valsartan in comparison to enalapril ($p < 0.001$, 1 week). The significant differences among treatment groups for each biomarker were sustained at 8 weeks. In an exploratory multivariable adjusted analysis of HF-rehospitalization or cardiovascular death, the concentrations of hsTnT, sST2 at week 1 were found to be significantly associated with subsequent outcome.

Conclusion: Biomarkers of myocardial stress are increased in ADHF patients and associated with outcome. As compared to enalapril, sacubitril/valsartan decreases hemodynamic stress and myocardial injury that is reflected by biomarkers, with an onset apparent within 1–4 weeks.

*Redrafted abstract

COMMENT

The PARADIGM study demonstrated the efficacy of sacubitril/valsartan in reducing the cardiovascular death or hospitalization for heart failure (HF) in patients with chronic heart failure with reduced ejection fraction (HFrEF). PIONEER-HF adds more vital information on the drugs efficacy in patients stabilized during hospitalization for acute decompensated heart failure (ADHF). In these patients, tolerance of the drug, ability to escalate the dose after in-hospital initiation, clinical and biomarker response are aspects that require more specific information.

The PIONEER-HF sub-study discusses the early- and near-term effects of initiation of sacubitril/valsartan versus enalapril on mechanistic biomarkers comprising hsTnT, soluble suppression of tumorigenicity 2 (sST2), and cGMP and NT-proBNP among patients with ADHF who are hemodynamically stabilized.

Stretched myocytes induce and release sST2; it reflects ventricular wall stress. This novel biomarker in various smaller studies has proved its worth as a prognostic marker in ADHF.

It is concluded by PIONEER-HF that patients who had higher baseline concentrations of hsTnT, sST2, and NT-proBNP were at higher absolute risk of rehospitalization for HF or cardiovascular death. The consecutive achieved concentrations during follow-up were found to be associated with subsequent rehospitalization for HF or cardiovascular death.

ARTICLE 4

Urinary Sodium Profiling in Chronic Heart Failure to Detect Development of Acute Decompensated Heart Failure

Martens P, Dupont M, Verbrugge FH, et al. Urinary sodium profiling in chronic heart failure to detect development of acute decompensated heart failure.
JACC Heart Fail. 2019;7(5):404-14.

*Abstract**

Objectives: We aimed to evaluate the association between urinary sodium (U_{Na}) concentration and pathophysiologic interaction with development of the acute heart failure (AHF) hospitalization.

Background: There is a lack of data on the longitudinal dynamics of U_{Na} concentration in chronic heart failure (HF) patients, comprising its temporal relationship with AHF hospitalization.

*Redrafted abstract

Methods: This study included stable, chronic HF patients who had either reduced or preserved ejection fraction; they were prospectively included for undergoing prospective collection of the morning spot U_{Na} samples for 30 consecutive weeks. For assessing the longitudinal changes in U_{Na} concentration, linear mixed modeling was used. Patients were followed for development of clinical endpoint of the AHF.

Results: Total 80 chronic HF patients were included in the study. Mean age of the patients was 71 ± 11 years; N-terminal pro-B-type natriuretic peptide (NT-proBNP) concentration was 771 ng/L (interquartile range: 221–1,906 ng/L); left ventricular ejection fraction (LVEF) was $33 \pm 7\%$. These patients prospectively submitted weekly prediuretic first void morning U_{Na} samples for 30 weeks. Total 1,970 U_{Na} samples were collected; mean U_{Na} concentration was 81.6 ± 41 mmol/L. Excretion of sodium remained stable over time on a population level (time effect, p = 0.663). However, interindividual differences showed presence of high [88 mmol/L U_{Na} (n = 39)] and low [73 mmol/L U_{Na} (n = 41)] sodium excreters. Only young age was found to be an independent predictor of high sodium excretion [odds ratio (OR) 0.91; 95% confidence interval (CI) 0.83–1.00; p = 0.045 per year)]. During follow-up period of 587 ± 54 days, 21 patients were admitted for AHF. Patients who developed AHF were observed to have significantly lower U_{Na} concentrations [$F_{(1.80)}$ = 24.063; p <0.001]. The discriminating capacity of U_{Na} concentration for detecting AHF persisted after inclusion of NT-proBNP and estimated glomerular filtration rate (eGFR) measurements as random effects (p = 0.041). Moreover, U_{Na} concentration decreased in the week preceding the hospitalization.

Furthermore, U_{Na} concentration dropped (U_{Na} = 46 ± 16 mmol/L vs. 70 ± 32 mmol/L, respectively; p = 0.003) in the week preceding the hospitalization and returned to the individual's baseline (U_{Na} = 71 ± 22 mmol/L, p = 0.002) following recompensation; whereas, such early longitudinal changes in dyspnea scores and weight were not apparent in the week preceding decompensation.

Conclusion: Overall, U_{Na} concentration was relatively stable over time, but large interindividual differences were present in stable, chronic HF patients. Patients who developed AHF had chronically lower U_{Na} concentration and had a further drop in concentration of U_{Na} during the week preceding hospitalization. Collection of ambulatory U_{Na} sample is feasible and can provide additional therapeutic and prognostic information.

COMMENT

Renal sodium retention is a likely marker of heart failure (HF) severity, and lower urinary sodium (U_{Na}) levels on diuretic therapy may correlate with decompensation in patients with HF and reduced ejection fraction. The utility of urine sodium as a novel biomarker has been highlighted in accompanying editorial in the same journal issue and takes us into the ability to use it in clinical practice.

As in hypertension research, U_{Na} excretion assessment will be more precise with 24 hours urine sodium concentrations for prediction of HF decongestant therapy and cardiovascular (CV) outcomes including recurrent hospitalization. The ease of estimating urine spot sodium cannot, however, be overlooked. Sodium and fluid retention being the hallmark of HF, this can be a frontline biomarker. Lower U_{Na}

concentrations typically reflect enhanced renal sodium retention in the context of a deficit in extracellular fluid (ECF) volume. Precautions are required before interpretation of the urine sodium results. Dose and type of diuretic agents being administered and the timing of the measurement in relation to diuretic administration should be considered as factors that also reduce or increase the urine volume.

ARTICLE 5

Utility of Cardiac Biomarkers in the Setting of Kidney Disease

Savoj J, Becerra B, Kim JK, et al. Utility of cardiac biomarkers in the setting of kidney disease. *Nephron. 2019;141(4):227-35.*

*Abstract**

Cardiovascular disease is prevalent in chronic kidney disease (CKD) patients and is responsible for nearly half of all deaths related with CKD. Unfortunately, the presence of CKD can result in challenging interpretation of cardiac biomarkers that are essential for accurate diagnosis and prompt management of heart failure (HF) and acute coronary syndrome. There is an increase in interest in new cardiac biomarkers, which may improve diagnostic accuracy reflecting myocardial injury, inflammation, and remodeling. It can be complicated to interpret these biomarkers in CKD because increase in levels may not reflect wall tension or myocardial injury but rather reduced urinary clearance with retention of solutes and/or overall chronic inflammation associated with CKD. In this review, the latest data on major and emerging cardiac biomarkers comprising of troponin, B-type natriuretic peptide, growth and differentiation factor-15, suppression of tumorigenicity 2, matrix gla protein (MGP), and galectin-3, and their diagnostic and prognostic utility in the CKD population was discussed.

COMMENT

Alterations in the cardiac biomarker levels with reduced kidney function have made acute coronary syndrome (ACS) diagnosis challenging. Chronic kidney disease (CKD) patients presenting with acute chest pain have non-ST elevation myocardial infarction (NSTEMI) more than twice as often as patients with normal kidney function. Elevation

*Redrafted abstract

in levels of biomarkers can be because of reduced urinary clearance or possibly chronic inflammation associated with CKD.

The hs-cTnT and hs-cTnI at 0 and 1 hour after are sensitive in ruling out NSTEMI in patients with CKD with estimated glomerular filtration rate (eGFR) less than 60 mL/min/1.73 m^2, and with lower specificity to rule-in disease was found to be lower as compared to patients with normal kidney function.

As per recommendations by the National Academy of Clinical Biochemistry Practice guidelines, a change in troponin level more than 20% within 6–9 hours as diagnostic for acute myocardial infarction (MI) in patients who have advanced CKD (eGFR <15 mL/min/1.73 m^2) but the cutoff levels for CKD stage I–III have been less defined.

There is an increase in N-terminal pro-B-type natriuretic peptide (NT-proBNP)/BNP ratios when eGFR falls below 30 mL/min/1.73 m^2. If eGFR is less than 60 mL/min/1.73 m^2, a NT-proBNP value more than 1,200 ng/L is considered best for exclusion of HF with lesser cutoff levels for further decrease of GFR. The soluble suppression of tumorigenicity 2 (sST2), in contrast to BNP and NT-proBNP, is not affected by the degree of kidney insufficiency among CKD patients with acute HF.

Emerging biomarkers like growth differentiation factor-15 (GDF-15), sST2, MGP, and galectin-3 have limited in patients with decreased eGFR. Galectin-3 levels are inversely and significantly related to eGFR, independent of left ventricular ejection fraction or HF.

ARTICLE 6

Temporal Patterns of 14 Blood Biomarker Candidates of Cardiac Remodeling in Relation to Prognosis of Patients with Chronic Heart Failure—The Bio-SHiFT Study

Bouwens E, Brankovic M, Mouthaan H, et al. Temporal patterns of 14 blood biomarker candidates of cardiac remodeling in relation to prognosis of patients with chronic heart failure—The Bio-SHiFT study. *J Am Heart Assoc. 2019;8(4):e009555.*

*Abstract**

Background: Remodeling biomarkers have high potential in predicting adverse events among chronic heart failure (CHF) patients. Temporal patterns during the course of CHF and particularly trajectory before an adverse event are, however, not known. In this study, authors studied prognostic value of the temporal patterns of 14 cardiac remodeling biomarker candidates among stable patients with CHF from the Bio-SHiFT (Serial Biomarker Measurements and New

*Redrafted abstract

Echocardiographic Techniques in Chronic Heart Failure Patients Result in Tailored Prediction of Prognosis) study.

Methods and Results: In total 263 CHF patients, trimonthly blood sampling during a median follow-up of 2.2 years was performed. For this analysis, all baseline samples were selected: two samples closest to the primary endpoint (PE), or last sample available for the endpoint-free patients. Therefore, in 567 samples, suppression of the galectin-3; galectin-4; tumorigenicity-2; matrix metalloproteinase-2, 3, and 9; growth differentiation factor-15; tissue inhibitor metallo-proteinase-4; aminopeptidase-N; perlecan; caspase-3; cystatin-B; cathepsin-D; and cathepsin-Z was measured. The PE was a composite of heart transplantation, cardiovascular mortality, HF hospitalization, and left ventricular assist device implantation. By joint modeling, associations between repeatedly measured biomarker candidates and the PE were investigated.

Median age of the patients was 68 (interquartile range 59–76) years; out of the total patients 72% were men; 70 patients reached the PE. Repeatedly measured suppression of galectin-3; galectin-4; tumorigenicity-2; matrix metalloproteinase-2 and 9; growth differentiation factor-15; perlecan; tissue inhibitor metalloproteinase-4; cathepsin-D; and cystatin-B levels were found to be significantly associated with the PE, and increased as the PE approached. Slopes of biomarker trajectories were also predictors of the clinical outcome, independent of their absolute level. Associations persisted after adjustment for pharmacological treatment and clinical characteristics. Suppression of tumorigenicity 2 was noted to be the strongest predictor (hazard ratio, 7.55 per SD difference, 95% CI 5.53–10.30), followed by growth differentiation factor-15 (4.06, 2.98–5.54), and matrix metalloproteinase-2 (3.59, 2.55–5.05).

Conclusion: In CHF patients, temporal patterns of remodeling biomarker candidates predict adverse clinical outcomes.

COMMENT

Suppression of tumorigenicity 2 (ST2), Gal-4, growth differentiation factor-15 (GDF-15), perlecan, and CSTB were the biomarkers at baseline to differentiate between patients who will reach the primary endpoint versus those who will remain event free. On serial estimation, ST2, GDF-15, and matrix metallo-proteinase-2 (MMP-2) were the strongest predictors of incident adverse clinical events. Temporal patterns and different rates of change of the marker were important predictors for implication in clinical practice.

Newer biomarkers carry incremental value for prediction of future CHF events in comparison to the established cardiac biomarkers NT-proBNP and hsTnT. Change in MMP-2, MMP-9, and TIMP-4 will be a new addition once established for prediction of incident events. Biomarkers that signal myocardial apoptosis, fibrosis, and hypertrophy like ST2 will find a prominent place in the flowchart of HF diagnostic assessment.

ARTICLE 7

Cardiovascular Biomarkers and Heart Failure Risk in Patients with Stable Atherothrombotic Disease: A Nested Biomarker Study from TRA 2°P-TIMI 50

Berg D, Freedman B, Bonaca MP, et al. Cardiovascular biomarkers and heart failure risk in patients with stable atherothrombotic disease: A nested biomarker study from TRA 2°P-TIMI 50.
J Am Coll Cardiol. 2019;73(9):257.

*Abstract**

Background: Patients who have stable atherothrombotic disease differ in their risk of developing heart failure (HF). Assessment of incident HF risk may be improved by circulating cardiovascular biomarkers.

Methods: The high-sensitivity troponin I (hsTnI) and brain natriuretic peptide (BNP) (Abbott ARCHITECT) were measured in 14,603 patients with prior myocardial infarction (MI), peripheral artery disease, or ischemic stroke, from the TRA 2°P-TIMI 50 trial, excluding those patients who had any prior HF or recent MI (<30 days). Using a priori cut-points, biomarkers were categorized. The HF endpoints were adjudicated retrospectively with blinded structured review of serious adverse events by using established definitions.

Results: The independent clinical risk predictors for HF included age 75 years or more, body mass index, hypertension, diabetes mellitus, prior peripheral artery disease, and prior cerebrovascular disease. Baseline hsTnI and BNP recognized a significant graded risk of HF independent of the clinical risk indicators, both individually (Fig. 1: left figure) and when considered together (Fig. 1: right figure). On adding to a multivariable Cox regression model with the clinical risk predictors (c-statistic 0.78), BNP (c-statistic 0.89), and hsTnI (c-statistic 0.83), each significantly improved the prognostic performance of the model (both p <0.001).

Conclusion: Biomarkers of the myocardial injury and hemodynamic stress (hsTnI and BNP) add to clinical risk indicators for incident HF risk prediction among patients who had stable atherothrombotic disease without prior HF.

*Redrafted abstract

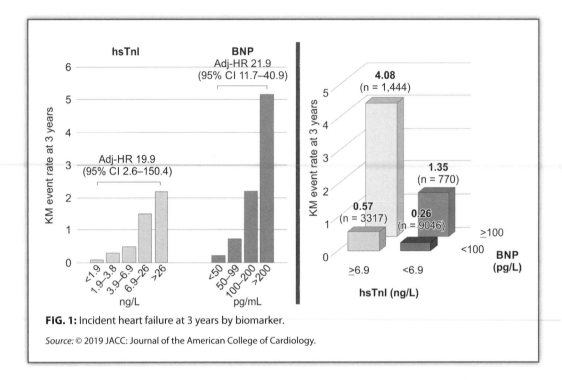

FIG. 1: Incident heart failure at 3 years by biomarker.

Source: © 2019 JACC: Journal of the American College of Cardiology.

COMMENT

Stable atherothrombotic disease spectrum has a significant burden of heart failure and often is under-evaluated in clinical practice. Serial echocardiography has not been able to make clinicians more vigilant. With this context, serial estimation of hs-troponin and BNP is value added to predict clinical heart failure. Pharmacotherapy may then target drugs which have protective mechanisms for heart failure.

Section 5

Imaging in Heart Failure in 2018

Section Editors: Jagdish Chander Mohan, Madhu Shukla, Vishwas Mohan

ARTICLE 1

Advances in Imaging and Heart Failure: Where are We Heading?

Adigopula S, Grapsa J. Advances in imaging and heart failure: Where are we heading?
Card Fail Rev. 2018;4(2):73-7.

*Abstract**

Following technological developments, advanced cardiac imaging has progressed significantly and it now works as a prognostic as well as a diagnostic tool. Constant follow-up with more advanced imaging such as stress imaging or baseline imaging such as echocardiography is the utmost requirement in heart failure patients. Imaging helps in offering better interventional procedures as well as treatment for the improvement of heart failure patients. The main aim of this review is to brief the newest imaging procedures in heart failure treatment and diagnosis.

COMMENT

Heart failure (HF) is a clinical syndrome of effort intolerance due to structural heart disease. Imaging is required in patients with HF for diagnosis, defining etiology, prognosis, therapy, and for serial evaluation for reversal or progression of pathophysiological processes (Flowcharts 1 and 2). Imaging, in simplest terms, separates heart failure with reduced ejection fraction (HFrEF) from non-HFrEF. Many imaging parameters have entered routine clinical practice for day-to-day management for greater diagnostic and prognostic precision. More emphasis is being placed on parametric imaging like 3D strain, tissue characterization by cardiac magnetic resonance imaging, molecular imaging, and other novel imaging modes. Change in tissue composition before change in cardiac function may allow early detection and intervention. In 2018, novel cardiac imaging studies have shown several unique aspects of cardiac performance, myocardial

*Redrafted abstract

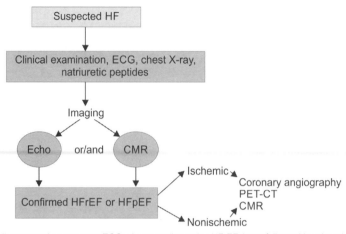

(CMR: cardiac magnetic resonance; ECG: electrocardiography; HFrEF: heart failure with reduced ejection fraction; HFpEF: heart failure with preserved ejection fraction; PET-CT: positron emission tomography-computed tomography)

FLOWCHART 1: Detailed schema of imaging in suspected heart failure (HF).

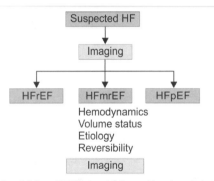

(HF: heart failure; HFrEF: heart failure with reduced ejection fraction; HFpEF: heart failure with preserved ejection fraction; HFmrEF: heart failure with midrange ejection fraction)

FLOWCHART 2: Imaging in routine clinical practice.

damage, and mechanisms of HF. This review summarizes some of these developments.

■ EXTRACELLULAR VOLUME, INFLAMMATION, AND HEART FAILURE

We have always been interested in searching a surrogate for invasive endomyocardial biopsy (EMB) for quantifying and characterizing the abnormal tissue in myocardium of HF patients. Native T1 and T2 mapping and gadolinium enhancement during cardiac magnetic resonance imaging have been at the forefront to claim that position. Estimation of extracellular matrix by a novel technique of combined use of native T1 mapping coupled with hematocrit measurement is an attractive biomarker. Extracellular volume (ECV) is defined as a coefficient of the changes in T1 in tissue and blood before and after contrast injection. ECV measured by this technique in normal persons is typically <25%. ECV has been touted as an estimate of diffuse fibrosis. ECV may contain inflammatory exudate, noninflammatory edema, diffuse fibrosis, and abnormal protein/nonprotein deposition. A recent study has attempted to clarify this issue.

Lurz et al. from Leipzig,[1] Germany studied and quantified ECV in 107 patients with suspected inflammatory cardiomyopathy who presented with recent onset HF. All had endomyocardial biopsy as a part of protocol. Myocardial inflammation (leukocyte >14/mm^2) was present in 66 patients. Despite similar ejection fraction and collagen volume content, ECV and T1 and T2 mapping values were greater in those with inflammation compared to those without inflammation. There was an excellent correlation between diffuse myocardial fibrosis by EMB and ECV in patients without inflammation. In true inflammatory cardiomyopathy, ECV, although expanded to a greater extent, was a poor predictor of myocardial fibrosis. This study confirms the value of ECV as an index of expanded extracellular matrix but not necessarily of diffuse myocardial fibrosis in nonischemic cardiomyopathies of recent onset. However, even long-standing nonischemic cardiomyopathies may have significant component of inflammation (Fig. 1). In some patients, microvascular dysfunction may increase noninflammatory edema. In these patients, ECV may be a marker of extent of disease but not necessarily a biomarker of extent of fibrosis or therapeutic success in serial studies.

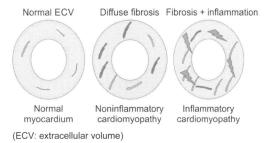

(ECV: extracellular volume)

FIG. 1: Schematic representation of myocardium in different states.

■ BODY FAT DISTRIBUTION AND TYPE OF HEART FAILURE

Subepicardial fat is a type of visceral fat deposited between myocardium and the pericardium and has pathophysiological links like visceral fat (Fig. 2). It has been estimated by transthoracic echocardiography, CT and magnetic resonance imaging. Its usual correlates are conventional risk factors for atherosclerosis. Visceral fat and inflammation are interlinked. Of late, there has been interest

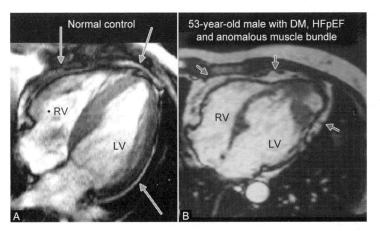

(DM: diabetes mellitus; HFpEF: heart failure with preserved ejection fraction; LV: left ventricle; RV: right ventricle)

FIG. 2: Steady-state free precession (SSFP) images of normal control (panel A) and that of diabetes with HFpEF, normal coronary angiogram and anomalous muscle bundles in the left ventricle. Note the greater amount of subepicardial fat in panel B (short arrows) compared to panel A (long arrows).

in subepicardial fat content and type of HF and its severity. Localized adiposity may produce local inflammation and mechanical dysfunction and may not be related to general adiposity. Subepicardial fat has been shown to be reduced or even normal in patients of HFrEF due to cardiac cachexia. Obesity is an important risk marker of heart failure with preserved ejection fraction (HFpEF). There have been speculations about subepicardial fat playing a role in pathogenesis of HFpEF especially in those with diabetes mellitus and even in those with midrange ejection fraction. Visceral fat including pericardial fat has been correlated with markers of inflammation and HbA1c. There has been an interesting work published on this aspect from University of Pennsylvania in 2018.

Chirinos et al.[2] studied the distribution and extent of fat and muscle mass by magnetic resonance imaging in various parts of body including subepicardial fat in 658 subjects. The study included normal subjects and those with both types of HF. Both types of HF were characterized by axial sarcopenia. However, subepicardial fat was increased only in HFpEF. The HFpEF patients had increased subcutaneous, visceral, and pericardial fat while HFrEF patients had reduced visceral and subcutaneous fat. The authors suggested that pericardial fat excites local inflammation, which plays a role in pathogenesis of HFpEF (Table 1).

DIABETES, ECHOCARDIOGRAPHY, AND INCIDENT HEART FAILURE

Of late, interest in diabetes and its relationship to HF has multiplied because of positive results of SGLT-2 inhibitors. Cardiac structural alterations are common in type 2 diabetes mellitus. These include diastolic dysfunction, left ventricular hypertrophy, left atrial enlargement, reduced global longitudinal strain, increased subepicardial fat, expanded ECV, nonischemic myocardial fibrosis, etc. However, it was not clear which of these is a better predictor of future HF. If we can identify the most significant morphological changes, we can take adequate preventive measures.

Wang et al.[3] studied 310 patients ≥65 years of age with type 2 diabetes mellitus with preserved ejection fraction and no ischemic heart disease by echocardiography. The most common abnormality was left atrial enlargement (35%), followed by left ventricular hypertrophy (23%), global longitudinal left ventricular strain <16% (23%), and grade 2 or more diastolic dysfunction (10%). Incident HF occurred in 11.2/100 patient-years. The only two independent parameters of prediction were left ventricular hypertrophy (odds ratio = 2.9) and global longitudinal strain <16% (odds ratio = 2.26). These high-risk patients may require a priori mineralocorticoid receptor antagonists, anti-renin–angiotensin therapy and SGLT-2 inhibitors. Further randomized

TABLE 1: Fat distribution in two types of heart failure (HF).

	HFrEF	HFpEF
Pericardial fat	Normal	Increased
Visceral fat	Reduced	Increased
Subcutaneous fat	Reduced	Increased

(HFrEF: heart failure with reduced ejection fraction; HFpEF: heart failure with preserved ejection fraction)

trials are needed to study the effect of cardioprotective agents in these patients.

■ NATURAL HISTORY OF ACUTE MYOCARDITIS

Acute myocarditis is suspected in patients presenting with recent onset of HF, atrioventricular blocks, ventricular arrhythmias, or chest pain like in acute coronary syndrome along with elevated biomarkers of cardiac injury and inflammation. Quite often, there are protean manifestations and diagnosis is missed. Acute myocarditis is a frequent cause of sudden death in young people. After diagnosis of myocarditis, its resolution is studied by serial decrease in inflammatory and cardiac biomarkers. Many patients with this entity slip into the phase of dilated cardiomyopathy following an acute episode while in many patients with nonischemic dilated cardiomyopathy, myocarditis is suspected. Natural history of myocarditis is of great interest but is poorly characterized.

In a large multicentric registry from Italy, Ammirati et al.[4] studied 443 patients (mean age 34 years) with proven myocarditis and followed these for a median of 3 years. In-hospital mortality was 3% and cardiac mortality and/or need for heart transplantation were 4% at 5 years. This study suggests relatively benign course of acute myocarditis. The most common symptom of presentation was acute chest pain (86%). About a quarter of all patients had complicated myocarditis (HF, arrhythmias, and atrioventricular blocks) while majority had uncomplicated course. Cardiac magnetic resonance (CMR) criteria of edema and nonischemic late gadolinium enhancement were used to diagnose acute myocarditis in 94% of all (Fig. 3). At follow-up, none of the patients in uncomplicated group had left ventricular ejection fraction <50% by CMR

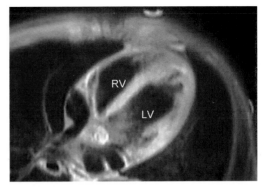

(LV: left ventricle; RV: right ventricle)

FIG. 3: T2-weighted short-tau inversion recovery (STIR) imaging on magnetic resonance showing generalized edema in a 23-year-old patient with acute myocarditis.

while in those with complicated hospital course, 14.5% had ejection fraction <50% on follow-up. From this study, it appears that patients who later on present with dilated cardiomyopathy are those who are admitted with some or the other complication in acute course. Dilated cardiomyopathy is rare in those cases of acute myocarditis who have an initial uncomplicated course. However, there are many unresolved issues. What about those patients who have positive late gadolinium enhancement on CMR on follow-up? Surely, those would be at high-risk. What is the proportion of patients with acute myocarditis who have evidence of myocardial damage on long-term follow-up?

■ CMR AS DIAGNOSTIC CRITERIA FOR CARDIAC SARCOIDOSIS

Cardiac sarcoidosis accounts for about 5% of total HF and significantly more reason for atrioventricular blocks and ventricular arrhythmias. Phenotype of isolated cardiac sarcoidosis is gaining more recognition as the cause of nonischemic segmental dysfunction. Its diagnosis lacks reliable and specific tools. Endomyocardial biopsy is rarely performed

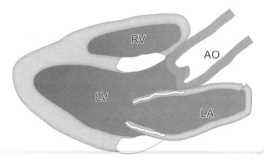

FIG. 4: Schematic diagram of the 3-chamber view showing characteristic sites for involvement in sarcoidosis.

and its yield is low because of patchy nature of the disease and also more basal involvement of the ventricles. Worldwide criteria proposed by the Japanese Ministry of Health are used, which are a combination of clinical and imaging parameters. CMR criteria are not given much weightage. Heart Rhythm Society in 2014 included specific patterns on CMR and positron emission tomography as major criteria. However, accuracy of CMR viz-a-viz criteria proposed by the Japanese Ministry of Health (the Gold standard) has not been adequately evaluated. There are very few causes of granulomatous inflammation and scarring of the basal left ventricular segments (Fig. 4) and hence CMR should stand pretty well as a diagnostic tool.

Jhang et al.[5] performed a meta-analysis of all studies published in the last 20 years on the subject in a total of 649 participants. Based upon the criteria used by the studies (no uniform criteria and no per-patient analysis), they found a sensitivity of 93% and specificity of 85% for CMR as compared to the prevalent gold standard. The results of this meta-analysis suggest that CMR could be used in the diagnosis of cardiac sarcoidosis and screening of the patients suspected with cardiac sarcoidosis. Other causes of granulomatous or inflammatory cardiomyopathies can be the confounders.

This study supports the inclusion of CMR findings as major criterion in this multi-system enigmatic granulomatous inflammatory cardiomyopathy. More exciting stuff for morphofunctional cartography is the fusion imaging combining fluorodeoxyglucose (FDG)-positron emission tomography with CMR, which is on the horizon.

■ SKELETAL MUSCLE BIOENERGETICS IN HF AND INTRAVENOUS IRON

Molecular imaging is, being increasing, used in studying pathogenesis and therapeutic success in HF. Magnetic resonance spectroscopy using ^{31}P has been deployed to estimate skeletal muscle inorganic phosphates, phosphocreatine, ATP, pH, etc. HF is characterized by reduced skeletal muscle mass, lower hemoglobin, higher natriuretic peptides, increased inorganic phosphates, and reduced ATP/inorganic phosphates and phosphocreatine/inorganic phosphates. These bioenergetics are further impaired during exercise compared to normal subjects. Iron deficiency in HF contributes to effort intolerance by way of reduced high-energy phosphate stores.

In a seminal study, Melenovsky et al.[6] studied skeletal muscle bioenergetics in patients with HF and the short-term effects of intravenous iron therapy in those patients with HF who had iron deficiency. They noted that skeletal myopathy was more pronounced in patients with HF and iron deficiency. Exercise-induced decrease in high energy phosphates and acidosis was accentuated in presence of iron deficiency and HF. However, 1 month after adequate iron supplementation, there was no change in high-energy phosphate content even though exercise capacity and iron stores showed significant improvement. This is because mitochondrial function restoration by iron replenishment may take more time or iron deficiency may be working through other mechanisms.

■ MALIGNANT LEFT VENTRICULAR HYPERTROPHY AND HFrEF

Left ventricular hypertrophy (LVH) is present in 10–15% of the adult population with or without hypertension. In the general population, physiological hypertrophy is rare. LVH may be associated with progressive myocyte loss and replacement fibrosis. It is necessary to find out which subjects with LVH are prone to future development of HF. Malignant LVH is the term used in epidemiologic studies for those patients who have evidence of LVH by CMR criteria along with above reference value of natriuretic peptides and/or cardiac troponin.

A recently published data[7] from Multi-Ethnic Study of Atherosclerosis (MESA) showed that malignant LVH was present in 7% of these middle-aged and elderly subjects free of cardiovascular disease at the time of initial CMR. Malignant LVH was associated with nearly 10-fold higher chance of developing HFrEF over a period of 12 years. Interestingly, men were at 32-fold higher risk of developing HFrEF, if they had malignant LVH on initial CMR examination. The study looked at only HFrEF occurrence and not HFpEF, which might occur more frequently.

■ LEFT ATRIAL RESERVOIR STRAIN AND HFrEF

Left atrium dilatation is common in HF. Patients with HF require multiparametric morphofunctional assessment for risk stratification and prognosis. Left atrial function is an important component of this strategy. Conventionally, left atrial volume index is recorded in comprehensive echocardiographic assessment of HF. It has been suggested that left atrial peak longitudinal reservoir strain is an easily measurable parameter of left atrial function with incremental value (Fig. 5). This parameter

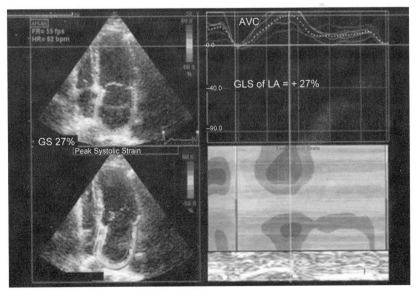

(GLS: global longitudinal strain)

FIG. 5: Peak global left atrial (LA) longitudinal strain of +27% in a patient with heart failure with reduced ejection fraction (HFrEF). *(For color version, see Plate 1)*

measures maximum left atrial lengthening during left ventricular systole. Its median value is about 40% and about twice of left ventricular longitudinal deformation. The two are tightly coupled in health but lose that tight relationship in disease. Left atrial function is significantly related to left ventricular systolic and diastolic dysfunction, but it has its own independent value. A recent study has corroborated this view.

Carluccio et al. evaluated the incremental prognostic utility of left atrial longitudinal strain in a consecutive series of 405 patients with HFrEF.[8] Peak left atrial longitudinal strain had significant relationship with left ventricular ejection fraction, severity of diastolic dysfunction left atrial volume, right ventricular systolic function, and left ventricular global longitudinal strain. However, the relationship of strain with left atrial volume was rather weak. After multivariable adjustments, peak left atrial longitudinal strain was the only independent negative predictor of all-cause mortality and rehospitalization. Future guidelines might include this parameter in the list of standard measurements in patients with HFrEF.

■ MYOCARDIAL FIBROSIS IN NEW-ONSET HF

Myocardial fibrosis, identified by late gadolinium enhancement cardiovascular magnetic resonance, predicts outcomes in chronic HF. Its incremental prognostic significance in new-onset HF and reduced left ventricular ejection fraction (LVEF) has not been studied. There is also the issue whether CMR should be routinely performed in all patients with new-onset HF (<6 months). Presence of myocardial fibrosis does not in any way change the guideline-mandated therapy, although it predicts poor prognosis.

Gulati et al.[9] evaluated the presence or absence and its extent of myocardial fibrosis by late gadolinium enhancement in a low-risk population of new-onset and apparently nonischemic HF. Long-term prognosis was related to the extent of myocardial fibrosis. About half of the patients had no myocardial fibrosis while the other half were almost equally divided between subendocardial and mid-myocardial fibrosis. All-cause and cardiovascular mortality was nearly three times higher with both types of fibrosis. However, at the moment, we have no additional therapy for patients with myocardial fibrosis.

■ STRESS IMAGING IN HFrEF

Stress imaging has been used to detect incipient HF by showing an inappropriate increasing in filling pressures. Stress imaging in patients with diagnosed HF may detect those having worse prognosis and hence requiring more aggressive therapy. Contractile reserve and preload reserve both can be studied by stress testing. Healthy hearts work on Frank–Starling principle wherein increase in preload improves contractility and stroke volume (Fig. 6). Frank–Starling mechanism may be still operative or blunted in HF.

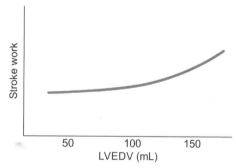

(LVEDV: left ventricular end-diastolic volume).

FIG. 6: Frank–Starling law of initial fiber stretch.

Matsumoto et al. studied the effect of preload increase by lower limb positive pressure compression on stroke work and left ventricular filling pressures by echocardiography in 120 patients with ambulatory HFrEF who were on optimal guidelines-mandated treatment.[10] A total of 23 normal controls were also studied. Preload increase by this method did not affect blood pressure or heart rate. There was an increase in preload in both groups as shown by increase in left ventricular end-diastolic volume and mitral Doppler early diastolic velocity. An increase in E/e' was noted in HF patients but not in normal controls. There was a blunted increase in stroke volume and stroke work in patients with HF (less than half of that in normal subjects). About 25% of the HF group showed a marked increase in E/e' (>30%) with no change in stroke work indicating absence of Frank–Starling compensation. On follow-up, these patients had adverse cardiac events. In well-compensated low-risk patients with HF, preload reserve and contractile reserve are coupled and intact. High-risk HFrEF patients have blunted contractile reserve in response to increase in preload. Absent diastolic and systolic contractile reserve identifies a high-risk group among HFrEF patients.

REFERENCES

1. Lurz JA, Luecke C, Lang D, et al. CMR–derived Extracellular Volume Fraction as a Marker for Myocardial Fibrosis: The Importance of Coexisting Myocardial Inflammation. JACC Cardiovasc Imaging. 2018;11(1):38-45.

2. Chirinos JA, Kim J, Goddam S, et al. Axial sarcopenia, subcutaneous, abdominal visceral and pericardial adiposity in heart failure with preserved and reduced ejection fraction. J Am Coll Cardiol. 2018;71(11):1205-338.

3. Wang Y, Yang H, Huyhn Q, et al. Diagnosis of Nonischemic Stage B Heart Failure in Type 2 Diabetes Mellitus: Optimal Parameters for Prediction of Heart Failure. JACC Cardiovasc Imaging. 2018;11(10):1390-400.

4. Ammirati E, Cipriani M, Moro C, et al. Clinical Presentation and Outcome in a Contemporary Cohort of Patients with Acute Myocarditis. Circulation. 2018;138(11):1088-99.

5. Jhang J, Li Y, Xu Q, et al. Cardiac Magnetic Resonance Imaging for Diagnosis of Cardiac Sarcoidosis: A Meta-Analysis. Can Respir J. 2018;2018:7457369.

6. Melenovsky V, Hlavata K, Sedivy P, et al. Skeletal Muscle Abnormalities and Iron Deficiency in Chronic Heart Failure. An Exercise 31P Magnetic Resonance Spectroscopy Study of Calf Muscle. Circ Heart Fail. 2018;11:e004800.

7. Peters MN, Seliger SL, Christenson RH, et al. "Malignant" Left Ventricular Hypertrophy Identifies Subjects at High Risk for Progression to Asymptomatic Left Ventricular Dysfunction, Heart Failure, and Death: MESA (Multi-Ethnic Study of Atherosclerosis). J Am Heart Assoc. 2018;7(4):e006619.

8. Carluccio E, Biagioli P, Mengoni A, et al. Left atrial reservoir function and outcome in heart failure with reduced ejection fraction: the importance of atrial strain by speckle tracking echocardiography. Circ Cardiovasc Imaging. 2018;11(11): e007696.

9. Gulati A, Japp AG, Raza S, et al. Absence of myocardial fibrosis predicts favourable long term survival in new-onset heart failure: A cardiovascular magnetic resonance study. Circ Cardiovasc Imaging. 2018;11(9):e007722.

10. Matsumoto K, Onishi A, Yamada H, et al. Noninvasive assessment of preload reserve enhances risk stratification of patients with heart failure with reduced ejection fraction. Circ Cardiovasc Imaging. 2018;11(5):e007160.

Section 6

Acute Heart Failure

Section Editors: K Venugopal, Vijay K Chopra

The Effect of Door-to-diuretic Time on Clinical Outcomes in Patients with Acute Heart Failure

Park JJ, Kim SH, Oh IY, et al. The effect of door-to-diuretic time on clinical outcomes in patients with acute heart failure. *JACC Heart Fail. 2018;6(4):286-94.*

Abstract*

Objective: This study was aimed at evaluating the impact of door-to-diuretic (D2D) time on mortality in patients who have acute heart failure (AHF) presenting to emergency department (ED).

Background: Majority of the patients with AHF presents with congestion. Their clinical outcomes can be improved by early decongestion with diuretic agents.

Methods: Total 5,625 consecutive patients hospitalized for AHF were enrolled in the Korea Acute Heart Failure registry. Those patients who received intravenous diuretic agents within 24 hours after ED arrival were included in the study. Early and delayed groups were described as those with D2D time 60 minutes or less and D2D time more than 60 minutes, respectively. The primary outcomes considered in the study were in-hospital death and postdischarge death at 1-month and 1-year based on the D2D time.

Results: The number of patients who met the inclusion criteria was 2,761. The median D2D time was 128 minutes (interquartile range, 63–243 min), and 24% (n = 663) patients were in the early group. Baseline characteristics were comparable between the groups. The rate of in-hospital death was comparable between the groups (5.0% vs. 5.1%; p >0.999), as well as the postdischarge 1-month (4.0% vs. 3.0%, log-rank p = 0.246) and 1-year (20.6% vs. 19.3%; log-rank p = 0.458) mortality rates. For each patient, Get With the Guidelines-Heart Failure risk score was calculated. In multivariate analyses with adjustment for Get With the Guidelines-Heart Failure risk score and other significant clinical covariates and propensity-matched analyses, D2D time was found to be not associated with clinical outcomes.

Conclusion: The D2D time was observed to be not associated with clinical outcomes in a large prospective cohort of patients who have AHF and presenting to an ED.

---

*Redrafted abstract

COMMENT

Door-to-balloon time has been a game changer in the management of ST elevation myocardial infarction (STEMI) with primary angioplasty. It has been clearly demonstrated that a shorter door-to-balloon time reduces mortality and morbidity in STEMI patients and guidelines have incorporated specific time windows for primary percutaneous coronary intervention (PCI). The authors in this article have tried to see whether a similar approach with earlier administration of diuretics intravenously would alter the outcomes in patients with acute decompensated heart failure (ADHF). This was a prospective cohort analysis of a registry data which included 2,761 patients. Early administration of intravenous diuretics within 60 minutes versus more than 60 minutes was compared. The D2D time was not associated with any favorable clinical outcomes. There was another similar study published in 2017 by Matsue et al. from Japan which demonstrated that earlier administration of diuretics in ADHF produced a 61% reduction in events which was a contrasting finding to the present study. There were some differences in the patient study groups but both were South-Asian population. The present study had a larger number of patients but the limitation was that it was not a randomized controlled trial and the timing and dose of diuretic therapy was not uniform. The differences in the findings of the two studies with opposite findings need to be examined.

ARTICLE 2

Frequency of Transition from Stage A to Stage B Heart Failure after Initiating Potentially Cardiotoxic Chemotherapy

Jones DN, Jordan JH, Meléndez GC, et al. Frequency of transition from stage A to stage B heart failure after initiating potentially cardiotoxic chemotherapy.
JACC Heart Fail. 2018;6(12):1023-32.

Abstract*

Objective: This study was aimed to evaluate the prevalence of American Heart Association/ American College of Cardiology Foundation (AHA/ACCF) heart failure (HF) stages after initiation of potentially cardiotoxic chemotherapy.

Background: In patients who receive potentially cardiotoxic chemotherapy, the frequency of transition from stage A to more advanced HF stages is not described properly.

*Redrafted abstract

Methods: Total 143 stage A HF patients with lymphoma and leukemia, breast cancer, renal cell carcinoma, or sarcoma were included. Blinded cardiac magnetic resonance measurements of left ventricular ejection fraction (LVEF) were obtained prior to and then at 3, 6, and 12–24 months after potentially cardiotoxic chemotherapy was initiated (Fig. 1).

Results: Three months after initiation of potentially cardiotoxic chemotherapy, 18.9% of patients transitioned from stage A to stage B HF. Total 83% and 80% of patients who had stage A HF at 3 months, respectively, exhibited stage A HF at 6 and 12–24 months; 68% and 56% of patients with stage B HF at 3 months, respectively, exhibited stage B HF at 6 and 12–24 months (p <0.0001 and p = 0.026, respectively).

Conclusion: Three months after initiation of potentially cardiotoxic chemotherapy, transitioning from stage A to stage B or remaining in stage A HF relates to longer-term (6–24 months post-treatment) assessments of HF stage.

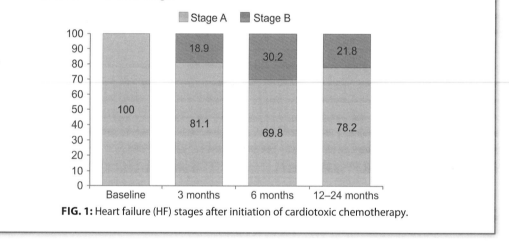

FIG. 1: Heart failure (HF) stages after initiation of cardiotoxic chemotherapy.

COMMENT

This is an interesting study. It is well recognized that a significant number of patients who receive chemotherapy for malignancy later develop cardiac toxicity and features of dilated cardiomyopathy. If an earlier diagnosis of transformation to heart failure can be demonstrated, it may prompt us to start guideline-based treatment for heart failure which may delay the progression of the disease process. The investigation that was used was cardiac MRI which is considered the gold standard in assessing left ventricular ejection fraction. Conventional 2D echocardiography may not pick up mild or earlier evidence of systolic heart failure. Strain imaging has been used in patients receiving chemotherapy to identify left ventricular dysfunction. A reduction of EF to 50% or a reduction of 10% from baseline were the criteria used to identify patient's transition from stage A to stage B. About 18.9% patients changed from stage A to stage B in 3 months time. About 83% patients in stage A at 3 months remained in stage A at 6 months and 80% at 12–24 months. Thus, patients receiving chemotherapy needs to be evaluated for transition from stage A to B at longer intervals up to 24 months.

ARTICLE 3

Randomized Evaluation of Heart Failure with Preserved Ejection Fraction Patients with Acute Heart Failure and Dopamine: The ROPA-DOP Trial

Sharma K, Vaishnav J, Kalathiya R, et al. Randomized evaluation of heart failure with preserved ejection fraction patients with acute heart failure and dopamine: The ROPA-DOP trial.
JACC Heart Fail. 2018;6(10):859-70.

*Abstract**

Objective: This study is aimed at comparing a continuous infusion diuretic strategy versus an intermittent bolus diuretic strategy, with addition of the low-dose dopamine (3 µg/kg/min) in the treatment of hospitalized patients who have heart failure with preserved ejection fraction (HFpEF).

Background: HFpEF patients when hospitalized with acute heart failure are prone to development of worsening renal function (WRF). However, inpatient treatment strategies for achieving safe and effective diuresis among HFpEF patients have not been carried out till date.

Methods: This was a prospective, randomized, clinical trial that included 90 HFpEF patients hospitalized with acute heart failure. These patients were randomized within 24 hours of admission to one of the four treatments: (1) intravenous bolus furosemide administered every 12 hours, (2) continuous infusion furosemide, (3) intermittent bolus furosemide with low-dose dopamine, and (4) continuous infusion furosemide with low-dose dopamine. Primary endpoint considered in the study was percent change in creatinine from baseline to 72 hours. Linear and logistic regression analyses were performed with tests for interactions between the diuretic and dopamine strategies.

Results: In comparison to intermittent bolus strategy, the continuous infusion strategy was found to be associated with higher percent increase in creatinine [continuous infusion: 16.01%, 95% confidence interval (CI) 8.58–23.45% vs. intermittent bolus: 4.62%, 95% CI 1.15–10.39%, $p = 0.02$]. There was no significant effect of low-dose dopamine on the percent change in creatinine (low-dose dopamine: 12.79%, 95% CI 5.66–19.92% vs. no dopamine: 8.03%, 95% CI 1.44–14.62%, $p = 0.33$). Continuous infusion was also observed to be associated with greater risk of WRF as compared to intermittent bolus [odds ratio (OR) 4.32, 95% CI 1.26–14.74, $p = 0.02$]. There were no differences in WRF risk with low-dose dopamine. There were no significant interaction observed between diuretic strategy and low-dose dopamine ($p > 0.10$).

Conclusion: In HFpEF patients hospitalized with acute heart failure, low-dose dopamine had no significant impact on renal function, and a continuous infusion diuretic strategy was associated with renal impairment.

[Diuretics and Dopamine in Heart Failure With Preserved Ejection Fraction (ROPA-DOP); NCT01901809].

*Redrafted abstract

COMMENT

Management of heart failure with preserved ejection fraction (HFpEF) presenting acutely has always been debated regarding optimum therapeutic strategies. Intravenous diuretics form the keystone of management but intermittent diuretic dose versus continuous infusion has always been debated. Low dose inotropic agents like dopamine have also been used in acute decompensated heart failure (ADHF) to potentiate the effects of intravenous diuretics. The ROPA-DOP study had two major observations. Low-dose dopamine did not worsen the renal function and a bolus dose intravenous furosemide was better than continuous infusion with respect to worsening renal function (WRF). The ROSE AHF trial 2013 showed that low-dose dopamine in patients with ADHF with preserved ejection fraction had a lower fluid and sodium output and increased mortality at 6 months and death or rehospitalizations at 2 months. ROPA-DOP study had four arms with and without low-dose dopamine and continuous versus intermittent bolus diuretic administration with the endpoint being WRF. The interesting observation was that the intermittent diuretic administration was associated with lower rates of worsening of renal function in patients with HFpEF. For physicians handling heart failure especially in India, it would be a great help to give intravenous bolus furosemide than to start on continuous infusion with inadequate staff and facilities. The use of low-dose dopamine has also not been advocated though this study did not show worsening of renal function compared to previous studies.

ARTICLE 4

Sudden Death in Heart Failure with Preserved Ejection Fraction and Beyond: An Elusive Target

Manolis AS, Manolis AA, Manolis TA, et al. Sudden death in heart failure with preserved ejection fraction and beyond: An elusive target.
Heart Fail Rev. 2019.

*Abstract**

Objective: This study evaluated the rates and predictors of sudden death (SD) or aborted cardiac arrest (ACA) in heart failure with preserved ejection fraction (HFpEF).

Background: Sudden death may be an important mode of death in HFpEF.

*Redrafted abstract

Methods: In this study, 1,767 patients who had HFpEF (EF ≥45%) enrolled in the Americas region of the Aldosterone Antagonist Therapy for Adults with Heart Failure and Preserved Systolic Function (TOPCAT) trial were studied. Independent predictors of composite SD/ACA were identified with stepwise backward selection by using competing risks regression analysis, which accounted for nonsudden causes of death.

Results: During a median 3.0-year (25th to 75th percentile: 1.9–4.4 years) follow-up, total 77 patients had SD/ACA, and 312 had non-SD/ACA. Corresponding incidence rates were 1.4 events/100 patient-years (25th to 75th percentile: 1.1–1.8 events/100 patient-years) and 5.8 events/100 patient-years (25th to 75th percentile: 5.1–6.4 events/100 patient-years). SD/ACA was lower but not statistically reduced in patients randomized to spironolactone: 1.2 events/100 patient-years (25th to 75th percentile: 0.9–1.7 events/100 patient-years) versus 1.6 events/100 patient-years (25th to 75th percentile: 1.2–2.2 events/100 patient-years). The subdistributional hazard ratio was 0.74 (95% confidence interval 0.47–1.16, p = 0.19). After accounting for competing risks of non-SD/ACA, insulin-treated diabetes mellitus (DM) and male sex were independently predictive of composite SD/ACA (C-statistic = 0.65). Covariates, which consist of eligibility criteria, age, coronary artery disease, left bundle branch block, ejection fraction, and baseline therapies, were not independently associated with SD/ACA. Sex and DM status were independent predictors in sensitivity analyses also, excluding patients who have implantable cardioverter-defibrillators and while predicting SD alone.

Conclusion: Sudden death was responsible for nearly 20% of deaths in HFpEF. Insulin-treated DM and male gender identified patients at higher risk for SD/ACA with modest discrimination. These data might guide SD preventative efforts in HFpEF in future.

[Aldosterone Antagonist Therapy for Adults With Heart Failure and Preserved Systolic Function (TOPCAT); NCT00094302].

COMMENT

Sudden cardiac death (SCD) and aborted cardiac arrest (ACA) are common modes of death in HFpEF in nearly 20% patients. This study was done in the Americas region of the TOPCAT trial. The purpose was to identify independent predictors of SCD and ACA in patients with HFpEF. Male sex and DM (insulin dependent) were independently predictive of SD/ACA. Age, EF, coronary artery disease left bundle-branch block (CAD LBBB), and treatment were not associated with independent predictive values. These two groups of patients may be candidates for ICD implantation. However, larger multicentric studies may be required to give a definite opinion on an expensive modality of treatment in those with HFpEF.

ARTICLE 5

Angiotensin–Neprilysin Inhibition in Acute Decompensated Heart failure

Velazquez EJ, Morrow DA, DeVore AD, et al. Angiotensin–neprilysin inhibition in acute decompensated heart failure
N Engl J Med. 2019;380(6):539-548.

Abstract*

In the United States, acute decompensated heart failure accounts for >1 million hospitalizations annually. It is still unknown whether initiation of sacubitril-valsartan therapy is safe and effective in patients hospitalized for acute decompensated heart failure.

Methods: Patients with heart failure with reduced ejection fraction (HFrEF) hospitalized for acute decompensated heart failure at 129 sites in the United States were enrolled in study. After hemodynamic stabilization, patients were randomized to receive either sacubitril-valsartan (target dose, 97 mg sacubitril plus 103 mg valsartan twice daily) or enalapril (target dose, 10 mg twice daily). The primary efficacy outcome considered in the study was the time-averaged proportional change in NT-proBNP (N-terminal pro-B-type natriuretic peptide) concentration from baseline level through weeks 4 and 8. Key safety outcomes were rates of worsening renal function, hyperkalemia, symptomatic hypotension, and angioedema.

Results: Out of total 881 patients who were randomly assigned, 440 received sacubitril-valsartan and 441 received enalapril. The time-averaged reduction in the concentration of NT-proBNP was significantly higher in the sacubitril-valsartan group as compared to the enalapril group. The ratio of the geometric mean of values obtained at weeks 4 and 8 to the baseline value was 0.53 in the sacubitril-valsartan group in comparison to 0.75 in the enalapril group [percent change, −46.7% vs. −25.3%; ratio of change with sacubitril-valsartan versus enalapril, 0.71; 95% confidence interval (CI) 0.63–0.81, $p < 0.001$]. The higher reduction in the concentration of NT-proBNP with sacubitril-valsartan as compared to that with enalapril was evident as early as week 1 (ratio of change, 0.76; 95% CI 0.69–0.85). The rates of worsening renal function, hyperkalemia, symptomatic hypotension, and angioedema were not significantly different between the two groups.

Conclusion: In patients with HFrEF hospitalized for acute decompensated heart failure, the initiation of sacubitril-valsartan therapy resulted in a higher reduction in the NT-proBNP concentration as compared to enalapril therapy. Rates of worsening renal function, hyperkalemia, symptomatic hypotension, and angioedema did not showed significant difference between the two groups.

(Funded by Novartis; PIONEER-HF ClinicalTrials.gov number, NCT02554890.)

*Redrafted abstract

COMMENT

Development of sacubitril-valsartan combination for heart failure management has been one of the most significant developments in heart failure therapy in recent years. The major studies on sacubitril-valsartan have been on patients with chronic heart failure (PARADIGM-HF) with reduced ejection fraction. The drug received FDA clearance for all cases of HFrEF class 2–4. It has also been studied in HFpEF (PARAGON-HF trial) but the results were not too satisfactory and failed to reach statistical significance. The present trial has studied the effect of sacubitril-valsartan in acute decompensated heart failure. This was a multicentric study in USA looking at the change in NT-proBNP and safety outcomes of hypotension, hyperkalemia, worsening of renal function, and angioedema. All patients were stabilized hemodynamically and then randomized to sacubitril-valsartan or enalapril as in the PARADIGM-HF trial. There was a greater reduction in the sacubitril-valsartan arm compared to the enalapril arm with no differences significant in the safety endpoints. One important aspect of the study was that 30% of the trial patients were Afro-Americans. The study gives the message that sacubitril-valsartan combination can be started in hospital in patients who present with acute heart failure who are hemodynamically stable and did not require inotropic support. Though the study population was fairly large, the results need to be replicated in larger populations in registries.

ARTICLE 6

Rivaroxaban in Patients with Heart Failure, Sinus Rhythm, and Coronary Disease

Zannad F, Anker SD, Byra WM, et al. Rivaroxaban in patients with heart failure, sinus rhythm, and coronary disease. *N Engl J Med. 2018;379(14):1332-42.*

*Abstract**

Background: Heart failure (HF) is related with thrombin-related pathways activation that predicts poor prognosis. Hypothesis in this study was that treatment with rivaroxaban, a factor Xa inhibitor, can lead to reduction in thrombin generation and improvement in outcomes for patients who have worsening chronic HF and underlying coronary artery disease.

*Redrafted abstract

Methods: This was a double-blind, randomized trial. Total 5,022 patients with chronic HF, a left ventricular ejection fraction of ≤40%, coronary artery disease, and increased plasma concentrations of natriuretic peptides and those not having atrial fibrillation were randomized to receive either rivaroxaban at a dose of 2.5 mg twice daily or placebo along with standard care after treatment for an episode of the worsening HF. The primary efficacy outcome considered in study was composite of death from any cause, stroke, or myocardial infarction. Fatal bleeding/bleeding into a critical space with potential for causing permanent disability was the principal safety outcome.

Results: The primary endpoint occurred in 25.0% (n = 626) of 2,507 patients assigned to rivaroxaban and in 26.2% (n = 658) of 2,515 patients assigned to placebo [hazard ratio (HR), 0.94, 95% confidence interval (CI) 0.84–1.05, p = 0.27] over a median follow-up period of 21.1 months. There was no significant difference in all-cause mortality between the rivaroxaban group and the placebo group (21.8% and 22.1%, respectively; HR 0.98, 95% CI 0.87–1.10). The principal safety outcome occurred in 18 patients receiving rivaroxaban and in 23 patients receiving placebo (HR 0.80, 95% CI 0.43–1.49, p = 0.48).

Conclusion: Rivaroxaban (at a dose of 2.5 mg twice daily) was not associated with a significantly lower rate of myocardial infarction, stroke, or death as compared to placebo in patients who had reduced left ventricular ejection fraction, worsening chronic HF, no atrial fibrillation, and coronary artery disease.

(Funded by Janssen Research and Development; COMMANDER HF ClinicalTrials.gov number, NCT01877915.)

COMMENT

In patients with worsening of heart failure (HF) and in sinus rhythm addition of rivaroxaban in lower doses along with standard care was compared to placebo. The hypothesis was that inhibition of thrombin-related pathways by oral anticoagulation agents could result in better patient outcomes. The agent used was rivaroxaban in a low dose of 2.5 mg twice daily in this large trial of more than 5,000 patients. The primary endpoints were death, MI or stroke and the safety endpoint was bleeding. There was no significant benefit of adding rivaroxaban in patients receiving standard care for worsening HF and sinus rhythm. One limitation highlighted was that in the absence of monitoring subclinical atrial fibrillation (AF) could have been missed. The main mechanisms of worsening and rehospitalization in HF seem to be unrelated to thrombin-mediated mechanisms and that could explain the lack of benefit of the newer oral anticoagulants like rivaroxaban.

ARTICLE 7

Influenza Vaccine in Heart Failure

Modin D, Jørgensen ME, Gislason G, et al. Influenza vaccine in heart failure.
Circulation. 2019;139(5):575-86.

*Abstract**

Background: In patients with heart failure (HF), influenza infection is considered to be a serious event. There is scarcity of knowledge regarding the association between influenza vaccination and outcome in HF patients. This study was aimed to evaluate whether influenza vaccination is associated with improvement in long-term survival among newly diagnosed HF patients.

Methods: This was a nationwide cohort study that included patients above 18 years of age and diagnosed with HF in Denmark between January 1, 2003 and June 1, 2015 (n = 134,048). Linked data were collected by using nationwide registries. In time-dependent Cox regression, vaccination status, number, and frequency during follow-up were treated as time-varying covariates.

Results: Follow-up was 99.8%. Median follow-up for all-cause death was 3.7 years (interquartile range 1.7–6.8 years). During the study period, the vaccination coverage of the study cohort was in the range of 16–54%. In unadjusted analysis, receiving one vaccination or more during follow-up was found to be associated with a higher risk of death. After adjustment for comorbidities, inclusion date, household income, education level, and medications receiving one vaccination or more was observed to be associated with 18% reduced risk of death (all-cause: hazard ratio (HR) 0.82, 95% CI 0.81–0.84, p <0.001; cardiovascular causes: HR 0.82, 95% CI 0.81–0.84, p <0.001). Greater cumulative number of vaccinations, annual vaccination, and vaccination early in the year (September–October) were associated with larger reductions in the risk of death in comparison to intermittent vaccination.

Conclusion: Among patients who had HF, after extensive adjustment for confounders, influenza vaccination was noted to be associated with a reduced risk of both the all-cause death and the cardiovascular death. Vaccination earlier in the year and frequent vaccination were associated with greater reductions in the risk of death in comparison to intermittent and late vaccination.

Clinical Perspective

What is New?
- At present, there is paucity of knowledge regarding the effect of influenza vaccination on survival in patients of HF.
- This study evaluated the association between influenza vaccination and survival in a large, nationwide cohort of unselected HF patients.

**Redrafted abstract*

- This study is the largest cohort study that has examined outcomes after influenza vaccination in HF patients.

What are the Clinical Implications?
Present study suggests that influenza vaccination can improve outcome in HF patients. As this was an observational study, results must be replicated in randomized clinical trials before making final conclusion.

COMMENT

A total of 50% of heart failure (HF) worsening causing acute decompensation and hospitalization is thought to be due to respiratory infections particularly influenza infections. Vaccination for influenza virus and pneumococcal infections are now being advocated to prevent rehospitalizations in patients with HF as well as COPD. This is a long-term study done in Denmark for 12 years which demonstrated that influenza vaccination improved outcomes in patients with HF significantly. Currently, there are no definite guidelines regarding the role of vaccination in patients with HF. There are no randomized controlled trials. Timely seasonal administration and frequent administration (annual) resulted in significant reductions in endpoints. This is a relatively inexpensive modality of treatment in patients with HF to prevent or reduce acute worsening in relatively stable patients.

ARTICLE 8

Bio-adrenomedullin as a Marker of Congestion in Patients with New-onset and Worsening Heart Failure

Ter Maaten JM, Kremer D, Demissei BG, et al. Bio-adrenomedullin as a marker of congestion in patients with new-onset and worsening heart failure.
Eur J Heart Fail. 2019;21(6):732-43.

*Abstract**

Background: Secretion of the adrenomedullin (ADM) is stimulated by volume overload for maintaining endothelial barrier function. In heart failure (HF), higher levels of biologically active (bio-) ADM are a counteracting response to vascular leakage and tissue edema.

*Redrafted abstract

Aim: To establish the value of plasma bio-ADM as a marker of congestion among patients who have worsening HF.

Methods and Results: The association of plasma bio-ADM levels with clinical markers of congestion, and its prognostic value was assessed in 2,179 patients who had new-onset or worsening HF enrolled in BIOSTAT-CHF (A systems BIOlogy Study to TAilored Treatment in Chronic Heart Failure) trial. In a separate cohort of 1,703 patients, data were validated. Patients who had higher plasma bio-ADM levels were old in age, had more severe HF, as well as had more signs and symptoms of congestion (all p <0.001). Out of 20 biomarkers, bio-ADM was found to be strongest predictor of clinical congestion score (r^2 = 0.198). In multivariable regression analysis, higher bio-ADM levels were observed to be associated with more edema, higher fibroblast growth factor 23, and higher body mass index. In hierarchical cluster analysis, bio-ADM was clustered with orthopnea, rales, edema, jugular venous pressure, and hepatomegaly. Higher bio-ADM levels were found to be independently associated with impairment in uptitration of angiotensin-converting enzyme (ACE) inhibitors/angiotensin receptor blockers (ARBs) after 3 months, but not of beta-blockers. Higher bio-ADM was independently associated with enhanced risk of the all-cause mortality as well as HF hospitalization (hazard ratio 1.16, 95% confidence interval 1.06–1.27, p = 0.002, per log increase). Analyses in the validation cohort resulted in similar findings.

Conclusion: Plasma bio-ADM levels in patients who have new-onset and worsening HF is associated with more severe HF and more orthopnea, edema, jugular venous pressure, and hepatomegaly. Thus, it is postulated in study that bio-ADM is a congestion marker that may be useful for guiding decongestive therapy.

COMMENT

Adrenomedullin (ADM) is a peptide hormone produced by endothelial cells and vascular smooth muscles and maintains the endothelial barrier. Disruption of the ADM system results in vascular leakage, systemic and pulmonary congestion. ADM levels are increased in sepsis and ADHF. Estimation of bio-ADM may be used to guide therapy with diuretics in pulmonary and systemic edema. The BIOSTAT-CHF trial had 2,179 patients. The greater levels were seen in older patients with more severe HF and were associated with clinical features of edema, orthopnea, hepatomegaly, and elevated jugular venous pressure (JVP). Higher levels were associated with increased all-cause mortality and hospitalizations. Previous clinical and preclinical studies have shown beneficial effects of ADM in myocardial infarction reduction, cardiac apoptosis, left ventricular (LV) remodeling, and aldosterone levels. Adrecizumab, a monoclonal antibody can combine with ADM and act as a therapeutic target in HF management. ADM may become a marker as well as therapeutic agent in HF management in future.

ARTICLE 9

Long-term Safety of Intravenous Cardiovascular Agents in Acute Heart Failure: Results from the European Society of Cardiology Heart Failure Long-term Registry

Mebazaa A, Motiejunaite J, Gayat E, et al. Long-term safety of intravenous cardiovascular agents in acute heart failure: Results from the European Society of Cardiology Heart Failure Long-term Registry. *Eur J Heart Fail. 2018;20(2):332-341.*

*Abstract**

Aim: This study was aimed to evaluate long-term safety of intravenous cardiovascular agents, such as inotropes, vasodilators, and/or vasopressors, in acute heart failure (AHF) patients.

Methods and Results: The European Society of Cardiology Heart Failure Long-term (ESC-HF-LT) registry was a prospective, observational registry conducted across 21 countries. Total 6,926 patients who had unscheduled hospitalizations for AHF were included. Out of these, 18.8% (n = 1,304) patients received a combination of intravenous (IV) diuretics and vasodilators, 12% (n = 833) patients received IV vasopressors and/or inotropes. Primary endpoint considered in this study was long-term all-cause mortality; main secondary endpoints were in-hospital and postdischarge mortality. No association was showed by adjusted hazard ratio (HR) between the use of IV vasodilator and diuretic and long-term mortality [HR 0.784, 95% confidence interval (CI) 0.596–1.032] nor in-hospital mortality (HR 1.049, 95% CI 0.592–1.857) in the matched cohort (n = 976 paired patients). On the contrary, adjusted HR showed a detrimental association between the use of IV vasopressor and/or inotrope and long-term all-cause mortality (HR 1.434, 95% CI 1.128–1.823), as well as in-hospital mortality (HR 1.873, 95% CI 1.151–3.048) in the matched cohort (n = 606 paired patients). There was no association between the use of IV vasopressors and/or inotropes and long-term mortality in patients discharged alive (HR 1.078, 95% CI 0.769–1.512). There was a detrimental association with vasopressors and/or inotropes noted in all geographic regions and, in catecholamines, dopamine was found to be associated with the highest risk of death (HR 1.628, 95% CI 1.031–2.572 vs. no inotropes).

Conclusion: There was no association of vasodilators with long-term clinical outcomes whereas, vasopressors and/or inotropes were found to be associated with increase in risk of all-cause death, mostly related to excess of in-hospital mortality.

**Redrafted abstract

COMMENT

European Society of Cardiology Heart Failure Long-term registry examined prospectively the long-term effects of intravenous drugs commonly used in heart failure namely vasodilators, diuretics, inotropes and vasopressors. Out of the 6,926 patients, 18.8% received IV vasodilators and diuretics, 12% received inotropes or vasopressors. Long-term all-cause mortality was the primary endpoint. The use of vasodilators and diuretics in the initial management did not affect the primary endpoints but vasopressors/inotropes were associated with increased long-term risk of all-cause mortality and cardiovascular mortality. These findings are in agreement with previous trials which showed that inappropriate use of inotropes/vasopressors were detrimental. Though, the use of inotropes and vasopressors has decreased, their use should only be in those with shock and evidence of severe tissue hypoperfusion. Another interesting observation was that dopamine had a greater mortality compared to dobutamine or levosimendan.

ARTICLE 10

Outcomes Associated with a Strategy of Adjuvant Metolazone or High-dose Loop Diuretics in Acute Decompensated Heart Failure: A Propensity Analysis

Brisco-Bacik MA, Ter Maaten JM, Houser SR, et al. Outcomes associated with a strategy of adjuvant metolazone or high-dose loop diuretics in acute decompensated heart failure: A propensity analysis.
J Am Heart Assoc. 2018;7(18):e009149.

*Abstract**

Background: In patients with acute decompensated heart failure (HF), increasing loop diuretic dose or adding a thiazide diuretic (when diuresis is not adequate) is recommended by guidelines.

Aim: To evaluate adverse events associated with a diuretic strategy that rely on high-dose loop diuretics or metolazone.

Methods and Results: In a propensity-adjusted analysis of all-cause mortality, patients who were admitted to three hospitals using a common electronic medical record with an HF discharge diagnosis who received intravenous loop diuretics were studied. Secondary outcomes considered

*Redrafted abstract

in study were hypokalemia (potassium <3.5 mEq/L), hyponatremia (sodium <135 mEq/L), and worsening renal function (a 20% or more reduction in estimated glomerular filtration rate). Out of 13,898 admissions, 7.5% (n = 1,048) patients used adjuvant metolazone. After the covariate and propensity adjustment, there was a strong association of metolazone with hypokalemia, hyponatremia, and worsening renal function (p <0.0001 for all) with minimal effect attenuation. After multivariate and propensity adjustment, metolazone remained associated with increased mortality [hazard ratio (HR) = 1.20, 95% confidence interval (CI) 1.04–1.39, p = 0.01]. High dose of loop diuretics were associated with hyponatremia and hypokalemia (p <0.002), but only worsening renal function remained significant (p <0.001) after propensity adjustment. After multivariate and propensity adjustment, high-dose loop diuretics were not associated with reduced survival (HR = 0.97 per 100 mg of IV furosemide, 95% CI 0.90–1.06, p = 0.52).

Conclusion: In acute decompensated HF, metolazone was found to be independently associated with hyponatremia, hypokalemia, worsening renal function, and increase in mortality after controlling for propensity to receive the metolazone and baseline characteristics. However, in similar experimental conditions, high-dose loop diuretics were not found to be associated with hyponatremia, hypokalemia, or reduced survival. Latest findings suggest that until it is proved by randomized controlled trial data, uptitration of loop diuretics can be a preferred therapeutic option as compared to routine early addition of thiazide-type diuretics when diuresis is not adequate.

COMMENT

In acute heart failure, there is a problem of inadequate diuresis and clinical deterioration. It is often a practice to use other diuretics with a different mode of action along with loop diuretics for increasing urine output. Metolazone is a commonly used drug in this situation. In the present study, two strategies were used—one to increase dose of loop diuretics and the other to add metolazone to intravenous loop diuretics. This is commonly practiced in our setting also. The study has clearly shown an increase in the primary endpoint of all-cause mortality and secondary endpoints of hypokalemia, hyponatremia, and worsening of renal function. An increase in dose of loop diuretics may be a better therapeutic option than adding metolazone when faced with inadequate diuresis.

Section 7

Chronic Heart Failure

Section Editors: Abraham Oomman, Vijay K Chopra

ARTICLE 1

Lower Hospitalization and Healthcare Costs with Sacubitril/Valsartan versus Angiotensin-converting Enzyme Inhibitor or Angiotensin-receptor Blocker in a Retrospective Analysis of Patients with Heart Failure

Albert, NM, Swindle JP, Buysman EK, et al. Lower hospitalization and healthcare costs with sacubitril/valsartan versus angiotensin-converting enzyme inhibitor or angiotensin-receptor blocker in a retrospective analysis of patients with heart failure.
J Am Heart Assoc. 2019;8(9):e011089.

*Abstract**

Background: In patients with heart failure with reduced ejection fraction (HFrEF), treated with sacubitril/valsartan (SAC/VAL), outcomes data are mainly limited to results of clinical trials. In this study, hospitalization and healthcare costs in real-world patients who had (HFrEF) treated with SAC/VAL versus angiotensin-receptor blocker or angiotensin-converting enzyme (ARB/ACE) inhibitor were compared.

Methods and Results: Stable patients with HFrEF who were treated with SAC/VAL or ARB/ACE inhibitor from October, 2015 to June, 2016 were identified by using retrospective administrative claims data. In propensity-matched cohorts, postindex hospitalization and healthcare costs were evaluated by using robust variance estimation. By using unadjusted Kaplan–Meier estimates and multivariable models, time to first hospitalization was modeled. Postindex all-cause healthcare costs were modeled by using an adjusted multivariable model. In 279 patients per matched cohort, postindex hospitalization risk was lower for SAC/VAL in comparison with ARB/ACE inhibitor by using Kaplan–Meier estimation and unadjusted Cox models. For HF hospitalization, the hazard ratio (HR) 0.56, 95% confidence interval (CI) 0.33–0.94, p = 0.030. Adjusted results were found to be comparable to unadjusted.

*Redrafted abstract

Mean (SD) monthly healthcare costs were lower for SAC/VAL as compared to ARB/ACE inhibitor for all of the categories except pharmacy, with hospital costs being specifically disparate between cohorts: for HF hospitalization, $248 ($1,588) for SAC/VAL versus $1,122 ($7,290) for ARB/ACE inhibitor. The adjusted risk of incurring increased all-cause postindex costs was lower for SAC/VAL as compared to ARB/ACE inhibitor [cost ratio (CR) 0.74, 95% CI 0.59–0.94, $p = 0.013$].

Conclusion: In clinical practice, patients having HFrEF treated with SAC/VAL were less likely to be hospitalized as compared to matched patients treated with ARB/ACE inhibitor. In spite of higher pharmacy costs, patients treated with SAC/VAL incurred lower monthly medical and total healthcare costs.

COMMENT

Even though there has been a revolutionary increase in the armamentarium against heart failure (HF), there has been no proportional improvement in the HF mortality and rehospitalizations. Lack of implementation of guideline-directed therapy (GDT) is a major cause of this disparity. Cost is a major barrier for uptake of new therapies like angiotensin receptor-neprilysin inhibitor (ARNI).

The real-world analysis in this study showed that HF with reduced ejection fraction (HFrEF) patients treated with ARNI had less risk of hospitalization and had less expenditure, i.e. total healthcare costs than those treated with angiotensin-receptor blocker or angiotensin-converting enzyme (ARB/ACE) inhibitor. This study complements the results of PARADIGM-HF, where SAC/VAL was superior to enalapril for reducing cardiovascular death and first HF

hospitalization. Data on real-world evidence on longitudinal health economic outcomes among patients with HFrEF who were treated with ARNI is scanty.

This paper showed that although combined and patient-paid outpatient pharmacy costs were higher for SAC/VAL compared with ARB/ACE inhibitor, this was offset by lower hospital costs and total healthcare costs in the SAC/VAL cohort.

The major economic burden of HF is incurred due to hospitalizations. By reducing hospitalizations, the overall cost can be reduced. The message to practitioners, patients, and health administers is to look at cost-effectiveness than the pill cost.

In the real world, treatment of HFrEF patients with ARNI may not only improve clinical outcomes but also reduce the long-term economic burden.

ARTICLE 2

Effects of Sacubitril/Valsartan on Physical and Social Activity Limitations in Patients with Heart Failure: A Secondary Analysis of the PARADIGM-HF Trial

Chandra A, Lewis EF, Claggett BL, et al. Effects of sacubitril/valsartan on physical and social activity limitations in patients with heart failure: A secondary analysis of the PARADIGM-HF trial.
JAMA Cardiol. 2018;3(6):498-505.

*Abstract**

Importance: In comparison to patients with other chronic diseases, health-related quality of life (HRQOL) of patients having heart failure (HF) is markedly decreased. This shows substantial limitations in social and physical activities. In Prospective Comparison of ARNI with an ACE inhibitor to Determine Impact on Global Mortality and Morbidity in Heart Failure (PARADIGM-HF) trial, sacubitril/valsartan improved overall HRQOL in comparison with enalapril, as determined by the Kansas City Cardiomyopathy Questionnaire (KCCQ).

Objective: To evaluate the impact of sacubitril/valsartan on social and physical activities.

Methods: The PARADIGM-HF trial was a randomized, double-blind, active treatment-controlled clinical trial, which was conducted between December 8, 2009 and March 31, 2014. Total 8,399 patients having New York Heart Association class II to IV disease and a left ventricular ejection fraction ≤40% at 1,043 centers in 38 countries were included. Between August 1, 2017 and December 25, 2017, data analysis was done. Patients either received sacubitril/valsartan 200 mg twice daily or enalapril 10 mg twice daily.

The HRQOL assessments were completed by patients by using KCCQ at the time of randomization, at 4 month, at 8 month, and at annual visits. The impact of sacubitril/valsartan on the components of the social and physical limitation sections of the KCCQ at 8 months and longitudinally as well as associated biomarkers and clinical outcomes were evaluated.

Results: At baseline, out of 8,399 patients, 90.7% (n = 7,618) completed the initial KCCQ assessment. Mean (SD) age of the patients was 64 (11) years; 78.6% (n = 5,987) were males and 21.4% (n = 1,631) were females. At baseline, patients reported greatest limitations in sexual relationships and jogging. Patients who received sacubitril/valsartan had significantly better adjusted change scores in most of the social and physical activities at 8 months and during 36 months in comparison with those who were receiving enalapril.

Largest improvement over enalapril was reported in sexual relationships (adjusted change score difference 2.72, 95% CI 0.97–4.46, p = 0.002) and household chores (adjusted change

*Redrafted abstract

score difference, 2.35; 95% CI 1.19–3.50; p <0.001); both remained through 36 months [overall change score difference 1.69, (95% CI 0.78–2.60), p <0.001; and 2.36 (95% CI 1.01–3.71), p = 0.001, respectively].

Conclusion: In patients who have heart failure with reduced ejection fraction (HFrEF), sacubitril/valsartan showed significant improvement in nearly all KCCQ social and physical activities as compared to enalapril; largest responses were noted in sexual relationships and household chores. Along with decreased likelihood of HF hospitalization, all-cause mortality, and cardiovascular death, sacubitril/valsartan may improve limitations in common activities among these patients.

COMMENT

Quality of life is as important as the quantity of life especially in elderly populations with heart failure with reduced ejection fraction (HFrEF). Heart failure (HF) patients have a poor quality of life comparable to kidney failure patients undergoing hemodialysis.

The PARADIGM-HF trial showed that sacubitril/valsartan as compared to enalapril significantly reduced HF-associated hospitalization, cardiovascular mortality, and all-cause mortality in patients with HFrEF; it also showed improvement in overall health-related quality of life (HRQOL) among surviving patients, as determined by the Kansas City Cardiomyopathy Questionnaire (KCCQ).

As compared with patients who received enalapril at the prespecified principal efficacy time point of 8 months, patients who were randomized to receive sacubitril/valsartan had greater change score differences in majority of the KCCQ social and physical activities, with the greatest adjusted change score difference observed in limitations of the sexual relationships. There was no significant difference observed in the overall difference in change score for social and physical limitations among patients treated with sacubitril/valsartan as compared to a difference of approximately 9 years in aging. A 5-point change in KCCQ overall score corresponds to 112 meter change in 6 minute walking distance and 2.5 mL/kg/min change in peak oxygen consumption (VO_2) in HFrEF patients. A 5-point decrease in KCCQ overall score indicates a deterioration in the patient's condition even if the patient is not overtly symptomatic.

In spite of comparison with an active treatment and that the baseline HRQOL was measured after an active run-in period with sacubitril/valsartan up to 6 weeks, the magnitude of improvement observed at 8 months after randomization in the PARADIGM-HF trial was similar to the HRQOL improvement observed with cardiac resynchronization therapy.

ARTICLE 3

Renal Effects and Associated Outcomes during Angiotensin-neprilysin Inhibition in Heart Failure

Damman K, Gori M, Claggett B, et al. Renal effects and associated outcomes during angiotensin-neprilysin inhibition in heart failure.
JACC Heart Fail. 2018;6(6):489-98.

*Abstract**

Objective: This study was aimed at evaluating the renal effects of sacubitril/valsartan among patients with heart failure and reduced ejection fraction (HFrEF).

Background: In patients with HFrEF, renal function is usually impaired; there may be further deterioration in renal function after blockade of the renin–angiotensin system.

Methods: In the Prospective Comparison of ARNI with an ACE inhibitor to Determine Impact on Global Mortality and Morbidity in Heart Failure (PARADIGM-HF) trial, total 8,399 patients who had HFrEF were randomly assigned to either sacubitril/valsartan or enalapril. For all patients, the estimated glomerular filtration rate (eGFR) was available. Urine albumin-to-creatinine ratio (UACR) was available in 1,872 patients at the time of screening, randomization, and at fixed time intervals during follow-up. Impact of study treatment on change in the eGFR and UACR, as well as on the renal and cardiovascular outcomes, according to eGFR and UACR, was evaluated.

Results: At the time of screening, the eGFR was 70 ± 20 mL/min/1.73 m^2 and 33% patients (n = 2,745) had chronic kidney disease. Median UACR was 1.0 mg/mmol [interquartile range (IQR): 0.4–3.2 mg/mmol] and 24% had a raised UACR. The reduction in eGFR during follow-up was less in sacubitril/valsartan group in comparison with enalapril [1.61 mL/min/1.73 m^2/year; (95% confidence interval (CI) 1.77–1.44 mL/min/1.73 m^2/year) vs. 2.04 mL/min/1.73 m^2/year (95% CI 2.21–1.88 mL/min/1.73 m^2/year), p <0.001] in spite of a greater increase in UACR with sacubitril/valsartan as compared to enalapril [1.20 mg/mmol (95% CI 1.04–1.36 mg/mmol) vs. 0.90 mg/ mmol (95% CI 0.77–1.03 mg/mmol), p <0.001]. The impact of sacubitril/valsartan on HF hospitalization or cardiovascular death was not modified by eGFR, UACR (p interaction = 0.70 and 0.34, respectively), or by change in the UACR (p interaction = 0.38).

Conclusion: In comparison to enalapril, sacubitril/valsartan resulted in a slower rate of reduction in the eGFR and improvement in cardiovascular outcomes, even among patients who had chronic kidney disease, in spite of causing a modest increase in the UACR.

*Redrafted abstract

COMMENT

One of the major reasons of the clinical inertia in initiating and uptitrating ARNI is the uncertainty of renal hemodynamics and its effects.

In this paper, it was evaluated whether slower rate of reduction in the eGFR with sacubitril/valsartan translated into reduction in end-stage renal disease or large decreases in the eGFR. Three components were included in the prespecified composite renal endpoint in PARADIGM-HF: (1) 50% or more reduction in the eGFR from baseline; (2) a more than 30 mL/min/1.73 m^2 reduction in the eGFR from baseline (and to less than 60 mL/min/1.73 m2); or (3) reaching end-stage renal disease.

As compared with enalapril, sacubitril/valsartan slowed the rate of reduction in the eGFR and had favorable effects on renal and cardiovascular outcomes in HFrEF patients with/without chronic kidney disease (CKD) and among those with/without microalbuminuria or macroalbuminuria. These renal and cardiovascular benefits were noted, although sacubitril/valsartan increased the UACR as compared with the enalapril.

This is potentially significant therapeutically as conventional renin–angiotensin–aldosterone system (RAAS) blockers are usually withdrawn or withheld in patients who have heart failure (HF) and renal dysfunction. Sacubitril/valsartan increased UACR in comparison with enalapril. Greater urinary albumin excretion has been observed to be associated with more rapid worsening of renal function in patients with CKD (though it is unknown if this is also true in HFrEF or not). This modest increase in UACR with ARNI stabilized over time and did not affect the cardiovascular benefits of treatment. In the enalapril treated patients, increase in UACR was associated with worse renal outcomes but not so in the ARNI group.

The RAAS inhibition is often associated with a transient decrease in eGFR in patients with HFrEF. This often results in premature discontinuation or lack of uptitration of these drugs in spite of clear evidence of cardiovascular benefits. In CHAMP-HF registry, there were higher rates of discontinuation or dose decreases (12%) for ARBs/ACE inhibitor than an initiation or dose increase (7%) at 12 months, resulting in lower rates of ARB/ACE inhibitor use at 12 months compared with baseline. Fear of worsening of eGFR and hypotension contributed mainly to this scenario. This study showed that reduction in eGFR was less in patients taking neprilysin inhibitor in addition to RAAS blocker, compared to RAAS blocker alone.

The translational implication of this study is that as ARNI had clinically significant benefits in spite of small increase in UACR, the renal mechanisms of action of neprilysin inhibition in heart failure merit specific studies.

ARTICLE 4

Sacubitril/Valsartan Reduces Ventricular Arrhythmias in Parallel with Left Ventricular Reverse Remodeling in Heart Failure with Reduced Ejection Fraction

Martens P, Nuyens D, Rivero-Ayerza M, et al. Sacubitril/valsartan reduces ventricular arrhythmias in parallel with left ventricular reverse remodeling in heart failure with reduced ejection fraction. *Clin Res Cardiol. 2019;108(10):1074-82.*

*Abstract**

Background: In the Prospective Comparison of ARNI with an ACE inhibitor to Determine Impact on Global Mortality and Morbidity in Heart Failure (PARADIGM-HF) trial, sacubitril/valsartan decreased the occurrence of sudden cardiac death (SCD). However, there is paucity of information about the mechanism.

Methods: In this study, patients of heart failure (HF) who received sacubitril/valsartan for a class-I indication equipped with an implantable cardioverter defibrillator (ICD) or cardiac resynchronization therapy (CRT) with remote telemonitoring were retrospectively analyzed. Device-registered arrhythmic events were determined {[ventricular tachycardia/fibrillation (VT/VF), appropriate therapy, nonsustained VT (NSVT): >4 beats and <30 s], hourly premature ventricular contraction (PVC) burden}, after initiation of sacubitril/valsartan (incident-analysis), and over an equal time period before initiation (antecedent-analysis).

Reverse remodeling to sacubitril/valsartan was defined as improvement in left ventricular ejection fraction (LVEF) of 5% or more between baseline and follow-up.

Results: Total 151 HF patients with reduced LVEF (29 ± 9%) were included. Patients were switched from ARB or ACE inhibitor to equal doses of sacubitril/valsartan (which were expressed as %-target-dose; before = 58 ± 30% vs. after = 56 ± 27%). Mean follow-up of both the incident and the antecedent analysis was 364 days. VT/VF burden dropped following the initiation (individual patients with VT/VF pre_n = 19 vs. post_n = 10, total episodes of VT/VF pre_n = 51 versus post_n = 14, both p <0.001), leading to reduction in occurrence of appropriate therapy (pre_n = 16 vs. post_n = 6; p <0.001). NsVT burden per patient also dropped (mean episodes pre_n = 7.7 ± 11.8 versus post_n = 3.7 ± 5.4; p <0.001). No impact on atrial fibrillation burden was noted. There was a significant drop in PVC burden that was associated with improvement in BiV pacing among patients with less than 90% biventricular (BiV) pacing at baseline. Higher degree of reverse remodeling was found to be associated with a lower burden of NSVT and PVCs (both p <0.05).

*Redrafted abstract

Conclusion: Sacubitril/valsartan initiation is associated with lower degree of VT/VF, which results in less ICD interventions. This beneficial effect on ventricular arrhythmias might be associated with cardiac reverse remodeling.

COMMENT

In Prospective Comparison of ARNI with an ACE inhibitor to Determine Impact on Global Mortality and Morbidity (PARADIGM), which was predominantly class II patients, even stable patients had a major annual event rate of 11% and one-third of them were unanticipated SCD. But the penetration of CRT/ICD in this group was not high. Even though valsartan–sacubitril showed significant benefit even in the CRT/ICD population, there was always a feeling that the numbers in this group were too low. In contradistinction to PARADIGM-HF population, the population in this study with very high class I recommended penetration of device therapy. This presented an interesting premise for investigating arrhythmia burden pre- and postinitiation of sacubitril/valsartan. In a regression meta-analysis, Shen et al. reported that over the past two decades, annual risk for SCD in HFrEF reduced from 6.5% to 3.3% by employment of guideline-directed HF pharmacotherapy. Valsartan–sacubitril forms the latest in the pharmacological armamentarium against SCD in HFrEF.

This study reported that there was a significant reduction in risk of ventricular arrhythmias and appropriate therapy after initiation of sacubitril/valsartan on CRT/ICD. Also, a hypothesis that this effect is mediated to some extent by beneficial left ventricular reverse remodeling, could be generated from the study. N-terminal pro-B-type natriuretic peptide (NT-proBNP) is decreased by sacubitril/valsartan that also decreases the echocardiographic presence of restrictive mitral filling pattern. A high level of NT-proBNP (which reflects the presence of increased wall stress) is an independent predictor of ventricular arrhythmias in HF.

In this study population, with a mean follow-up period of 364 days, the 1-year prevalence of appropriate therapy was 3.9% following initiation of sacubitril/valsartan [which is in the similar range of SCD as reported in the PARADIGM-HF (3.3% per year)]. Some of the cases of SCD might have been prevented in the PARADIGM-HF trial with a more robust background treatment of ICDs. However, our data also showed that with optimal pharmacotherapy implementation, the risk for developing a substrate for antitachycardia interventions by an ICD diminishes. This again re-emphasizes the importance of GDT of pharmacotherapy when considering ICD for primary prevention in HFrEF.

Another interesting aspect of this study was that even though the PV burden reduced after initiation of ARNI, the real reduction happened after achieving the maximum dose. This also points toward the importance of guideline-directed dose of ARNI in reducing events. There is a widespread tendency among clinicians not to uptitrate ARNI to maximum dose after initiation.

ARTICLE 5

Dapagliflozin and Cardiovascular Outcomes in Type 2 Diabetes

Wiviott SD, Raz I, Bonaca MP, et al. Dapagliflozin and cardiovascular outcomes in type 2 diabetes. *N Engl J Med. 2019;380(4):347-57.*

*Abstract**

Background: Dapagliflozin is a selective inhibitor of sodium-glucose cotransporter-2 (SGLT-2), which promotes glucosuria in patients with type 2 diabetes mellitus (T2DM). The cardiovascular safety profile of dapagliflozin is not defined.

Methods: Patients with T2DM, who had or were at risk for atherosclerotic cardiovascular disease, were randomly assigned to receive either dapagliflozin or placebo. The primary safety outcome considered in study was a composite of major adverse cardiovascular events (MACE), which was defined as myocardial infarction, ischemic stroke, or cardiovascular death. The primary efficacy outcomes included MACE and a combination of cardiovascular death or hospitalization for heart failure (HF). Secondary efficacy outcomes included a renal composite [40% or more decrease in estimated glomerular filtration rate (eGFR) to less than 60 mL/min/1.73 m^2 of body-surface area; new end-stage renal disease; or death from renal or cardiovascular causes] and death from any cause.

Results: Total 17,160 patients were evaluated. These included 10,186 patients without athero-sclerotic cardiovascular disease, followed for a median of 4.2 years. Primary safety outcome analysis revealed that dapagliflozin met the pre-specified criterion for noninferiority to placebo with regard to MACE [upper boundary of the 95% confidence interval (CI) <1.3; p <0.001 for noninferiority]. Two primary efficacy analyses showed that dapagliflozin did not result in a lower rate of MACE [8.8% in the dapagliflozin group and 9.4% in the placebo group; hazard ratio (HR) 0.93, 95% CI 0.84–1.03, p = 0.17], but it resulted in a lower rate of cardiovascular death or hospitalization for HF (4.9% vs. 5.8%; HR 0.83, 95% CI 0.73–0.95, p = 0.005), which reflected a lower rate of hospitalization for HF (HR 0.73; 95% CI 0.61–0.88). No between-group difference was noted in terms of cardiovascular death (HR 0.98, 95% CI 0.82–1.17). In the dapagliflozin group, renal event occurred in 4.3% patients and in 5.6% in the placebo group (HR 0.76, 95% CI 0.67–0.87); death from any cause occurred in 6.2% patients in dapagliflozin group and 6.6% in placebo group (HR 0.93, 95% CI 0.82–1.04). Diabetic ketoacidosis was observed to be more common with dapagliflozin as compared to placebo (0.3% vs. 0.1%, p = 0.02), as was the rate of genital infections that resulted in discontinuation of the regimen or that were considered as serious adverse events (0.9% vs. 0.1%, p <0.001).

*Redrafted abstract

Conclusion: In T2DM patients (who had or were at risk for atherosclerotic cardiovascular disease), treatment with dapagliflozin did not result in a higher or lower rate of MACE as compared to placebo; it resulted in a lower rate of cardiovascular death or hospitalization for HF, which reflects a lower rate of hospitalization for HF.

COMMENT

After EMPA-REG and CANVAS trials, cardiovascular outcomes with dapagliflozin were assessed in DECLARE–TIMI 58. It was a large trial involving more than 17,000 patients with a median of 4.2 years. In this period, the number who had MACE was more than 1,500 and the number who had cardiovascular deaths or hospitalization for HF was 900. One of the striking features of this trial was numbers without clinical atherosclerotic cardiovascular disease (more than 10,000 patients). EMPA-REG population was almost totally secondary prevention (established ARCVD) and CANVAS had two-thirds in secondary prevention category. In DECLARE study, two-thirds were primary prevention category (no established ARCVD). Most of the cardiovascular outcome trials concentrated on MACE. This study also brought into focus an important endpoint, i.e. hospitalization for HF. DECLARE data indicate that in the primary prevention cohort (patients with no established atherosclerotic cardiovascular disease), inhibition of SGLT-2 may prevent serious clinical events, especially hospitalization for HF, and may decrease the likelihood of renal disease progression.

In spite of focused collection of events, there was no evidence of a higher risk of amputations, fractures, or stroke with dapagliflozin as compared to placebo. Similarly, in spite of the observation of an excess of cases of bladder cancer in previous smaller studies of dapagliflozin, a lower rate of bladder cancer with dapagliflozin as compared to placebo was observed. The rate of diabetic ketoacidosis was higher in the dapagliflozin group as compared to placebo group, which is a finding that is consistent with findings in other SGLT-2 inhibitor studies.

There was no benefit with respect to cardiovascular death whereas this was shown in the EMPA-REG trial with empagliflozin. This could be due to the difference in the populations, especially prior myocardial infarction (MI).

The DECLARE study showed the efficacy and safety of dapagliflozin in a diabetic population in which the majority did not have clinical atherosclerotic vascular disease, which reflects the practice scenario.

ARTICLE 6

Comparison of the Effects of Glucagon-like Peptide Receptor Agonists and Sodium-glucose Cotransporter-2 Inhibitors for Prevention of Major Adverse Cardiovascular and Renal Outcomes in Type 2 Diabetes Mellitus: A Systematic Review and Meta-analysis of Cardiovascular Outcomes Trials

Zelniker TA, Wiviott SD1, Raz I, et al. Comparison of the effects of glucagon-like peptide receptor agonists and sodium-glucose cotransporter 2 inhibitors for prevention of major adverse cardiovascular and renal outcomes in type 2 diabetes mellitus.
Circulation. 2019;139(17):2022-31.

*Abstract**

Background: Sodium-glucose cotransporter-2 (SGLT-2) inhibitors and glucagon-like peptide-1 receptor agonists GLP-1 RA have appeared as two novel classes of antihyperglycemic agents, which also lower cardiovascular risk. The relative advantages in patients with/without established atherosclerotic cardiovascular disease (ASCVD) for different outcomes with these classes of drugs are still not defined.

Methods: This is a systematic review and trial-level meta-analysis of SGLT-2 inhibitors and GLP-1 RA cardiovascular outcomes trials using the EMBASE and PubMed databases. Primary outcomes included hospitalization for heart failure (HHF); the composite of myocardial infarction, stroke, and cardiovascular death [major adverse cardiovascular events (MACE)]; and progression of kidney disease.

Results: This study included data from eight trials and 77,242 patients. Out of total patients, 55.6% (n = 42,920) in GLP-1 RA trials and 44.4% (n = 34,322) in SGLT-2 inhibitors trials were included. Both classes of drug decreased MACE in a similar magnitude; GLP-1 RA reduced risk by 12% [hazard ratio (HR) 0.88, 95% confidence interval (CI) 0.84–0.94, p <0.001] and SGLT-2 inhibitors by 11% (HR 0.89, 95% CI 0.83–0.96, p = 0.001). For both of the drug classes, this treatment effect was observed to be restricted to 14% reduction in patients with established ASCVD (HR 0.86, 95% CI 0.80–0.93, p = 0.002), while no effect was observed among patients without established ASCVD (HR 1.01, 95% CI 0.87–1.16, p = 0.81; p-interaction 0.028). SGLT-2 inhibitors decreased HHF by 31% (HR 0.69, 95% CI 0.61–0.79, p <0.001), while GLP-1 RA did not have a significant effect (HR 0.93, 95% CI 0.83–1.04, p = 0.20). Both SGLT-2 inhibitors (HR 0.62, 95% CI 0.58–0.67, p <0.001) and GLP-1 RA (HR 0.82, 95% CI 0.75–0.89, p <0.001) decreased the risk of kidney disease

*Redrafted abstract

progression including macroalbuminuria. However, only SGLT-2 inhibitors lowered the risk of worsening eGFR, end-stage kidney disease, or renal death (HR 0.55, 95% CI 0.48–0.64, p <0.001).

Conclusion: GLP-1 RA and SGLT-2 inhibitors reduced atherosclerotic MACE to a comparable degree in patients with established ASCVD in studies reported to date, while SGLT-2 inhibitors had a more marked impact on HHF prevention and kidney disease progression. In the decision-making process, their distinct clinical benefit profiles should be considered when treating T2DM patients.

COMMENT

The agents reducing cardiovascular outcomes in diabetic patients are gaining importance and most guidelines emphasize this fact. GLP-1 RA and SGLT-2 inhibitors have been shown to reduce the risk of cardiovascular events in patients with type 2 diabetes mellitus (T2DM). However, the choice among them or the relative benefits of these in different patient populations has not been very clear. This meta-analysis showed that both GLP-1 RA and SGLT-2 inhibitors reduce the risk of MACE by approximately 14% in patients with known ASCVD. The risk of myocardial infarction (MI) and cardiovascular (CV) death was reduced by both drugs but only GLP-1 RA reduced the risk of stroke. However, SGLT-2 inhibitors robustly reduced the relative risk of HHF by 31%, whereas there was only a nonsignificant 7% relative risk reduction with GLP-1 RA.

The effects of both groups of drugs on renal events were different. GLP-1 RA mainly reduces macroalbuminuria. In diabetic kidney disease, albuminuria is a well-established biomarker for events. However, it is only a surrogate marker and may even be absent in patients with reduced eGFR. Reduction in eGFR has emerged as the more meaningful endpoint of greater importance. When macroalbuminuria is excluded, GLP-1 RA had nonsignificant relative reduction by 8%. This is in distinction to a recent meta-analysis of SGLT-2 inhibitors that showed robust relative risk reductions by 45% for the composite of reductions in eGFR, end-stage kidney disease, and death due to renal causes. The mechanism of action of these two drug classes is still not well elucidated. The HBA1c reductions by both drug classes are modest and hence their cardiovascular benefits may be nonglucose mediated through pleiotropic effects.

ARTICLE 7

Empagliflozin Ameliorates Adverse Left Ventricular Remodeling in Nondiabetic Heart Failure by Enhancing Myocardial Energetics

Santos-Gallego CG, Requena-Ibanez JA, San Antonio R, et al. Empagliflozin ameliorates adverse left ventricular remodeling in nondiabetic heart failure by enhancing myocardial energetics.
J Am Coll Cardiol. 2019;73(15):1931-44.

*Abstract**

Background: Cardiac benefits of empagliflozin, in the Empagliflozin Cardiovascular Outcome Event Trial in Type 2 Diabetes Mellitus Patients–Removing Excess Glucose (EMPA-REG OUTCOME) trial, cannot be described solely by its antihyperglycemic activity.

Objective: Hypothesis of this study was that cardiac benefits of empagliflozin are mediated by switching myocardial fuel metabolism away from glucose toward the ketone bodies (KB), which helps in improvement of myocardial energy production.

Methods: In this study, heart failure (HF) was induced in nondiabetic pigs (n = 14) by 2-hour balloon occlusion of proximal left anterior descending artery. Randomization of animals was done to either empagliflozin or placebo for 2 months. Evaluation of animals was done with three-dimensional echocardiography and cardiac magnetic resonance imaging. Analysis of myocardial metabolite consumption was done by simultaneous blood sampling from the coronary artery as well as coronary sinus. For molecular evaluation, myocardial samples were obtained. Animals with nonmyocardial infarction served as a comparison.

Results: Both groups had similar initial ischemic myocardial injury. However, empagliflozin group showed amelioration of adverse remodeling at 2 months [lower left ventricular (LV) mass, reduced LV dilatation, less LV sphericity] as compared to the control group. LV systolic function (echocardiography-derived strains and LV ejection fraction) was improved; neurohormonal activation was also improved. In comparison to nonmyocardial infarction, control animals enhanced myocardial glucose consumption largely through anaerobic glycolysis while decreasing utilization of branched-chain amino acid (BCAA) and free fatty acid (FFA). Pigs who were treated with empagliflozin did not consume glucose (decrease in myocardial glucose uptake, and glucose-related enzymes) but in its place switched toward use of FFA, KB, and BCAA (enhanced myocardial uptake of these three metabolites, and increased activity/expression of the enzymes implicated in the metabolism of FFA/KB/BCAA). Empagliflozin enhanced myocardial ATP content and increased myocardial work efficiency.

Conclusion: In a nondiabetic porcine model, empagliflozin ameliorates adverse cardiac remodeling and HF.

*Redrafted abstract

COMMENT

Mechanisms for CV benefits with SGLT-2 inhibitors are not clear. It may be multi-factorial, more due to pleiotropic actions than glucose lowering effects. The proposed mechanisms include hemodynamic effects, hormonal (glucagon, RAAS, NP) effects, hydroxybutyrate (beta), i.e. superfuel hypothesis, hydrogen exchanger inhibition (sodium), hemoglobin/hematocrit increase, hyperfiltration reduction (tubuloglomerular feedback), heart rate (no increase), hemorheology (improvement), hyperuricemia (reduction), and hepatic fat reduction [nonalcoholic fatty liver disease (NAFLD)].

This study was performed in nondiabetic porcine HF model. The first significant finding was that empagliflozin significantly improved adverse anatomical LV remodeling, reduced neurohormonal activation, and increased LV systolic function. Second significant finding was that these empagliflozin's cardiac benefits are mediated by switch in the myocardial fuel metabolism away from the low-yield energy-producing glucose metabolism toward FFA, KB, and BCAA, which enhances myocardial energy production.

This study points toward the benefits of SGLT-2 inhibitors in nondiabetic failing hearts.

ARTICLE 8

SGLT-2 Inhibitors for Primary and Secondary Prevention of Cardiovascular and Renal Outcomes in Type 2 Diabetes: A Systematic Review and Meta-analysis of Cardiovascular Outcome Trials

Zelniker TA, Wiviott SD, Raz I, et al. SGLT2 inhibitors for primary and secondary prevention of cardiovascular and renal outcomes in type 2 diabetes: a systematic review and meta-analysis of cardiovascular outcome trials. *Lancet. 2019;393(10166):31-9.*

Abstract*

Background: The magnitude of impact of sodium-glucose cotransporter-2 (SGLT-2) inhibitors on particular renal and cardiovascular outcomes and whether heterogeneity is based on the key baseline characteristics and is still not defined.

*Redrafted abstract

Methods: This is a systematic review and meta-analysis including randomized, placebo-controlled, cardiovascular outcome trials of SGLT-2 inhibitors among patients who had type 2 diabetes mellitus (T2DM). PubMed and Embase were searched for trials published up to September 24, 2018. A standardized data form was used to search and extract data, and any discrepancies were resolved by consensus. The efficacy outcomes included major adverse cardiovascular events (MACEs) (stroke, myocardial infarction, or cardiovascular death); composite of cardiovascular death or hospitalization for heart failure (HF); and renal disease progression. Hazard ratios (HRs) with 95% confidence intervals (CIs) were pooled across trials, and efficacy outcomes were stratified by baseline presence of HF, degree of renal function, and atherosclerotic cardiovascular disease.

Findings: Data was extracted from three identified trials and 34,322 patients (60.2% with atherosclerotic cardiovascular disease). There were 3,342 MACEs, 2,028 cardiovascular deaths or hospitalizations for HF events, and 766 renal composite outcomes. SGLT-2 inhibitors decreased MACEs by 11% (HR 0.89, 95% CI 0.83–0.96, p = 0.0014), with benefit seen only among patients who had atherosclerotic cardiovascular disease [0.86 (0.80–0.93)] and not in those without [1.00 (0.87–1.16); p for interaction = 0.0501]. SGLT-2 inhibitors decreased the risk of cardiovascular death or hospitalization for HF by 23% [0.77 (0.71–0.84), p <0.0001], with similar benefit among patients with/without atherosclerotic cardiovascular disease and with/without history of HF. SGLT-2 inhibitors decreased the risk of renal disease progression by 45% [0.55 (0.48–0.64), p <0.0001], with similar benefit in those with/without atherosclerotic cardiovascular disease. Magnitude of benefit of the SGLT-2 inhibitors varied with baseline renal function, with higher decrease in hospitalizations for HF (p for interaction = 0.0073) and lesser decrease in progression of renal disease (p for interaction = 0.0258) in patients who had more severe kidney disease at baseline.

Interpretation: The SGLT-2 inhibitors have moderate benefits on atherosclerotic MACEs, which appear confined to patients who have proven atherosclerotic cardiovascular disease. However, they have robust advantages on decreasing hospitalization for HF and progression of renal disease irrespective of existing atherosclerotic cardiovascular disease or history of HF.

RESEARCH IN CONTEXT

Evidence Before this Study: The SGLT-2 inhibitors have been studied in large cardiovascular outcome trials in patients who had T2DM and were proved to decrease the risk of cardiovascular events. Patients with established atherosclerotic cardiovascular disease as well as those with multiple risk factors but without the disease were evaluated in these trials.

The magnitude of benefit appeared to be greater, within individual trials, on MACEs in subgroups with proven atherosclerotic cardiovascular disease, though formal heterogeneity was not demonstrated. On the basis of these findings, American and European guidelines recommend use of SGLT-2 inhibitors for patients who have T2DM and atherosclerotic cardiovascular disease, independent of glucose control considerations.

However, due to the low number of patients and events in those patients with multiple risk factors alone, no single trial was sufficiently powered to test for such heterogeneity.

Once data from the DECLARE-TIMI 58 trial of dapagliflozin versus placebo became available, authors prospectively planned to meta-analyze cardiovascular outcome findings from the dedicated cardiovascular outcome trials stratified by presence/absence of proven atherosclerotic cardiovascular disease. PubMed and EMBASE were searched by using Medical Subject Heading terms such as "clinical trial", "T2DM", and "sodium-glucose cotransporter-2 (SGLT-2) inhibitor" for trials published up to September 24, 2018 to find all randomized cardiovascular outcome trials for SGLT-2 inhibitors.

Added Value of this Study: By incorporating data from DECLARE-TIMI 58 trial, EMPA-REG OUTCOME trial, and the CANVAS Program trial, the present meta-analysis of SGLT-2 inhibitors cardiovascular outcome trials demonstrated that the clinical benefit of SGLT-2 inhibitors in decreasing the risk of stroke, myocardial infarction, or cardiovascular death was present only in patients who had established atherosclerotic cardiovascular disease and not among those with multiple risk factors. In contrast, decreases in risk of hospitalization for HF or progression of renal disease were robust irrespective of presence of the atherosclerotic cardiovascular disease or HF at baseline.

Implications of All the Available Evidence: These data indicate that SGLT-2 inhibitors should be considered in patients who have T2DM irrespective of presence of the atherosclerotic cardiovascular disease or history of HF, provided that SGLT-2 inhibitors safely decrease HbA1c and decrease the risk of hospitalization for HF and progression of renal disease across a broad spectrum of patients with T2DM. Reductions in MACEs in patients with proven cardiovascular atherosclerotic disease can also be expected.

COMMENT

Even though we tend to divide the population into primary and secondary prevention categories, it is artificial and looks only at atherosclerotic risk factors and not the risk of hospitalization for HF or major renal events. The following risk factors were considered to be the strongest predictors for cardiovascular outcomes and death in diabetics: low physical activity, smoking, and glycated hemoglobin, systolic blood-pressure, and low-density lipoprotein (LDL) cholesterol levels outside the target ranges. Patients who had T2DM, with five risk-factor variables within target ranges, seemed to have little or no excess risks of myocardial infarction, stroke, and death in comparison with general population.

Having all five risk-factor variables within the target ranges could theoretically eliminate the excess risk of acute myocardial infarction. However, there was a substantial excess risk of hospitalization for HF among patients who had all the variables within target ranges. Subodh Verma in his editorial argued that this study, while providing a reminder of the triple threat of pump, pipes, and filter problems in T2DM, also provides compelling evidence that SGLT-2 inhibitors should now be considered as first-line therapy after metformin in most people with T2DM, irrespective of whether or not they have established atherosclerotic vascular disease, chronic kidney disease, or HF.

ARTICLE 9

Comparative Effectiveness of Canagliflozin, SGLT-2 Inhibitors and Non-SGLT-2 Inhibitors on the Risk of Hospitalization for Heart Failure and Amputation in Patients with Type 2 Diabetes Mellitus: A Real-world Meta-analysis of 4 Observational Databases (OBSERVE-4D)

Ryan PB, Buse JB, Schuemie MJ, et al. Comparative effectiveness of canagliflozin, SGLT2 inhibitors and non-SGLT2 inhibitors on the risk of hospitalization for heart failure and amputation in patients with type 2 diabetes mellitus: A real-world meta-analysis of 4 observational databases (OBSERVE-4D).
Diabetes Obes Metab. 2018;20(11):2585-97.

*Abstract**

Aims: For treatment of type 2 diabetes mellitus (T2DM), sodium-glucose cotransporter-2 (SGLT-2) inhibitors are indicated. Cardiovascular benefit is reported by some SGLT-2 inhibitors and below-knee lower extremity (BKLE) amputation by some of the studies. This study is aimed at evaluating the real-world comparative effectiveness within the SGLT-2 inhibitors class and compared with non-SGLT-2 inhibitors antihyperglycemic agents.

Materials and Methods: In this study, data was extracted from four large US administrative claims databases for characterizing risk and providing population-level estimates of effects of canagliflozin on hospitalization for heart failure (HHF) and BKLE amputation versus other SGLT-2 inhibitors and non-SGLT-2 inhibitors in patients of T2DM. Relative hazards of outcomes in all new users and a subpopulation with proven cardiovascular disease were examined by comparative analyses using a propensity score-adjusted new-user cohort design.

Results: In all the four databases (460,885 new users of non-SGLT-2 inhibitors, 142,800 new users of canagliflozin, 110,897 new users of other SGLT-2 inhibitors), the meta-analytic hazard ratio estimate for HHF with canagliflozin versus non-SGLT-2 inhibitors was 0.39 (95% CI 0.26–0.60) in on-treatment analysis. Estimate for BKLE amputation with canagliflozin versus non-SGLT-2 inhibitors was 1.01 (95% CI 0.93–1.10) in the intent-to-treat analysis and 0.75 (95% CI 0.40–1.41) in the on-treatment analysis. Effects in the subpopulation with established cardiovascular disease were comparable for both outcomes. There were no consistent differences between canagliflozin and other SGLT-2 inhibitors.

Conclusion: This large comprehensive analysis showed that canagliflozin and other SGLT-2 inhibitors demonstrated HHF benefits that were consistent with the clinical trial data, but showed no enhanced risk of BKLE amputation versus non-SGLT-2 inhibitors. In the subpopulation with established cardiovascular disease, HHF and BKLE amputation results were comparable. This study further helps in characterizing the potential benefits and harms of SGLT-2 inhibitors in routine clinical practice to complement evidence from previous observational studies and clinical trials.

*Redrafted abstract

COMMENT

The OBSERVE-4D is a large and comprehensive retrospective observational study comparing canagliflozin and other SGLT-2 inhibitors. After CANVAS publication, there were significant concerns of BKLE. This study has given direct head-to-head comparative evidence for BKLE amputation or HHF in individual drugs within the SGLT-2 inhibitors class.

A consistent pattern was reported by the analyses, which suggest a class effect of SGLT-2 inhibitors that decreases the risk of HHF relative to non-SGLT-2 inhibitors. Neither canagliflozin nor other SGLT-2 inhibitors demonstrated a consistently enhanced risk of BKLE amputation relative to non-SGLT-2 inhibitors in either the overall population or within the subpopulation of patients who had established cardiovascular disease, although none of the analyses was adequately powered for ruling out possibility of a modest effect.

This data offers some reassurance about the below knee limb amputations scare about canagliflozin. However, clinicians should use caution in using SGLT-2 inhibitors in patients with osteoporosis, prior amputations, severe peripheral artery disease (PAD), peripheral neuropathy or active lower extremity soft tissue ulcers or infections.

Section 8

Electrophysiology, Pacing and Ablation

Section Editor: Balbir Singh

ARTICLE 1

Outcome of Cardiac Sarcoidosis Presenting with High-grade Atrioventricular Block

Nordenswan HK, Lehtonen J, Ekström K, et al. Outcome of cardiac sarcoidosis presenting with high-grade atrioventricular block.
Circ Arrhythm Electrophysiol. 2018;11:e006145.

Abstract*

Background: Symptomatic high-grade atrioventricular block (AV block) is considered to be the most common as well as often the only presenting manifestation (lone AV block) of cardiac sarcoidosis. It is recommended to implant an intracardiac cardioverter defibrillator in place of a pacemaker. However, the true risk of fatal arrhythmia, one incident to the lone AV block specifically, is still known poorly.

Method: In this study, Myocardial Inflammatory Diseases in Finland Study Group Registry was used for analyzing the presentations, pacemaker therapy, left ventricular (LV) function, and ventricular arrhythmias in cardiac sarcoidosis. Total 325 cases of cardiac sarcoidosis were diagnosed from year 1988 to 2015 in Finland. Out of these, 143 patients presented with Mobitz II second degree or third degree AV block in absence of other explanatory cardiac disease. Mean age of the patients was 52 years; 112 patients were women.

Result: Concomitant with AV block at presentation, there were 20 patients with either severe LV dysfunction with ejection fraction less than 35% or ventricular tachycardia (VT) and 29 patients with nonsevere LV dysfunction (ejection fraction, 35–50%); whereas, 90 patients had AV block alone. During median follow-up of 2.8 years, 23 sudden cardiac deaths (SCD) (aborted or fatal) and 19 VT were recorded as arrhythmic endpoint events. The composite 5-year incidence (95% confidence interval) was found to be 56% (36–88%) in the AV block subgroup with VT or severe LV dysfunction as compared to 24% (12–49%) in the subgroup with nonsevere LV dysfunction and 24% (15–38%) with lone AV block (p = 0.019). The 5-year incidence of SCD was noted to be 34% (16–71%), 14% (6–35%), and 9% (4–22%) in the respective subgroups (p = 0.060).

Conclusion: The risk of SCD is significant in cardiac sarcoidosis presenting with high-grade AV block with/without LV dysfunction or VT. The consensus recommendation of implanting an intracardiac cardioverter defibrillator when permanent pacing is required appears to be well-founded.

---

*Redrafted abstract

COMMENT

In this study, 355 patients of sarcoidosis were included out of which 139 presented with high-grade atrioventricular block (AV block) needing a pacemaker; 49 also had ventricular arrhythmias or left ventricular ejection fraction (LVEF) <35% along with AV block. In rest 90, only AV block was present.

Risk of sudden death or ventricular tachycardia on follow-up	
Atrioventricular block with vent arrhythmia or low ejection fraction	56%
Atrioventricular block alone	24%

In conclusion, even though the risk of sudden cardiac death (SCD) and ventricular tachycardia (VT) is lower in the group of patients with AV block alone still is quite significant and warrants implantable cardioverter-defibrillator (ICD) as the first line therapy in patients with sarcoid and AV block.

ARTICLE 2

Catheter Ablation for Atrial Fibrillation with Heart Failure

Marrouche NF, Brachmann J, Andresen D, et al. Catheter ablation for atrial fibrillation with heart failure. *N Engl J Med. 2018;378:417-27.*

*Abstract**

Background: Mortality and morbidity are reported to be higher in patients with atrial fibrillation and heart failure as compared to those with heart failure alone. Catheter ablation for the atrial fibrillation has been suggested for improvement in outcomes in patients who have heart failure and are otherwise receiving suitable treatment.

Method: This study included patients who had symptomatic paroxysmal or persistent atrial fibrillation and did not responded to antiarrhythmic drugs, had unacceptable side effects, or were not willing to take these drugs. These patients were randomized to undergo either catheter ablation (n = 179) or medical therapy (rate/rhythm control) (n = 184) for atrial fibrillation along with guidelines-based therapy for heart failure. All of the patients had New York Heart Association (NYHA) class II, III, or IV heart failure, a left ventricular ejection fraction (LVEF) of ≤35%, and an implanted defibrillator. The primary endpoint considered in this study was a composite of death from hospitalization for worsening heart failure or any other cause.

Results: After median follow-up period of 37.8 months, the primary composite endpoint occurred in significantly lesser number of patients in the ablation group as compared to the medical therapy group [51 patients (28.5%) vs. 82 patients (44.6%), hazard ratio (HR), 0.62, 95% confidence interval (CI) 0.43–0.87, p = 0.007]. There were significantly lesser number of patients in the ablation group who died from any cause [24 (13.4%) vs. 46 (25.0%); HR 0.53, 95% CI 0.32–0.86, p = 0.01]; were hospitalized for worsening heart failure [37 (20.7%) vs. 66 (35.9%), HR 0.56, 95% CI 0.37–0.83, p = 0.004]; or died from cardiovascular causes [20 (11.2%) vs. 41 (22.3%), HR 0.49, 95% CI 0.29–0.84, p = 0.009].

Conclusion: Catheter ablation for atrial fibrillation among patients who had heart failure was associated with a significantly reduced rate of a composite endpoint of death from any cause or hospitalization for worsening heart failure as compared to the medical therapy.

COMMENT

Catheter Ablation versus Standard Conventional Treatment in patients with left ventricular dysfunction and Atrial Fibrillation trial (CASTLE-AF)

In this study, patients with paroxysmal or persistent atrial fibrillation, New York Heart Association (NYHA) class II to IV, left ventricular ejection fraction (LVEF) <35% and with an implantable cardioverter-defibrillator (ICD) were randomized to RF ablation or medical management (with good rhythm or rate control).

After a median follow-up of 37.8 months, catheter ablation was associated with reduction of the primary composite endpoint of death from any cause or hospitalization for worsening heart failure (HR 0.62, 95% CI 0.43–0.87, p = 0.007). Similarly, catheter ablation resulted in statistically significant reduction of the individual endpoints of all-cause mortality, hospitalization for worsening heart failure, and cardio-vascular death, compared with medical therapy. Catheter ablation was found to be associated with an improvement of LVEF by about 8%.

However, it must be acknowledged that a large majority of patients were excluded in the screening and selected patients considered good for ablation were randomized. So these results cannot be generalized and apply to select group of patients.

ARTICLE 3

Permanent His-bundle Pacing for Cardiac Resynchronization Therapy in Patients with Heart Failure and Right Bundle Branch Block

Sharma PS, Naperkowski A, Bauch TD, et al. Permanent His-bundle pacing for cardiac resynchronization therapy in patients with heart failure and right bundle branch block.
Circ Arrhythm Electrophysiol. 2018;11:e006613.

Abstract*

Background: In patients with left bundle branch block, left ventricular (LV) systolic dysfunction, and heart failure, cardiac resynchronization therapy (CRT) using biventricular pacing is considered to be an effective therapy. Among patients who have right bundle branch block (RBBB), benefits of biventricular pacing may be limited. Recently, permanent His bundle pacing (HBP) has been reported as an option for CRT. This study was aimed at assessing the feasibility and outcomes of HBP among patients who have RBBB and heart failure.

Method: In this study, HBP was attempted as a primary or rescue (failed LV lead implant) strategy among patients who had reduced left ventricular ejection fraction (LVEF), RBBB, QRS duration 120 ms or more, and New York Heart Association (NYHA) class II to IV heart failure. During follow-up, echocardiographic data, implant characteristics, and NYHA functional class were evaluated.

Results: Mean age of the patients was 72 ± 10 years; 15% of the patients were females. Patients had an average LVEF of $31 \pm 10\%$. HBP was successful in 95% (37 of 39) of the patients with narrowing of RBBB in 78% of the cases.

His capture and bundle branch block correction thresholds were noted to be 1.1 ± 0.6 V and 1.4 ± 0.7 V at 1 ms, respectively. During mean follow-up period of 15 ± 23 months, significant narrowing of QRS was observed from 158 ± 24 ms to 127 ± 17 ms ($p = 0.0001$), along with an increase in LVEF from $31 \pm 10\%$ to $39 \pm 13\%$ ($p = 0.004$) and improvement in NYHA functional class from 2.8 ± 0.6 to 2 ± 0.7 ($p = 0.0001$) with HBP. In three patients, increase in capture threshold occurred.

Conclusion: Among patients with RBBB and reduced LVEF, permanent HBP was found to be associated with significant narrowing of QRS duration and improvement in LV function. Permanent HBP seems to be a promising option for CRT among patients who have RBBB and reduced LVEF.

COMMENT

Right bundle branch block (RBBB) patients with LV dysfunction have not consistently shown benefit with cardiac resynchronization therapy (CRT) leading to confusion as to which of them should be selected for this therapy. Recently, His bundle permanent pacing has shown to recruit the normal conduction and produce a narrow QRS.

His bundle pacing was attempted as a primary or rescue (failed LV lead implant) strategy in patients with reduced left ventricular ejection fraction (LVEF), RBBB, QRS duration ≥120 ms, and New York Heart Association (NYHA) class II to IV heart failure.

His bundle pacing (HBP) was successful in 37 of 39 patients (95%) with narrowing of RBBB in 78% cases. During a mean follow-up of 15 ± 23 months, there was a significant narrowing of QRS from 158 ± 24 ms to 127 ± 17 ms ($p = 0.0001$), increase in LVEF fraction from $31 \pm 10\%$ to $39 \pm 13\%$ ($p = 0.004$), and improvement in NYHA functional class from 2.8 ± 0.6 to 2 ± 0.7 ($p = 0.0001$) with HBP.

This is the first study of HBP in patients with RBBB and LV dysfunction; this could be an exciting area for these patients and will lead to more patients benefiting.

*Redrafted abstract

Effect of Interventricular Electrical Delay on Atrioventricular Optimization for Cardiac Resynchronization Therapy

Gold MR, Yu Y, Singh JP, et al. Effect of interventricular electrical delay on atrioventricular optimization for cardiac resynchronization therapy.
Circ Arrhythm Electrophysiol. 2018;11(8):e006055.

Abstract*

Background: Routine atrioventricular optimization (AVO) is not reported to improve outcomes with the cardiac resynchronization therapy (CRT). However, recently, subgroup analyses of multicenter CRT trials have recognized electrocardiographic or lead positions to be associated with benefit from AVO. This analysis was aimed at evaluating whether the interventricular electrical delay modifies the effect of AVO on reverse remodeling with CRT.

Methods: In this substudy of the SMART-AV trial (SMARTDELAY Determined AV Optimization), 275 subjects were included. These were randomly assigned to either an electrogram-based AVO (SmartDelay) or nominal atrioventricular delay (120 ms). Interventricular delay was described as time between peaks of the right ventricular (RV) and left ventricular (LV) electrograms (RV-LV duration). CRT response was defined prospectively as more than 15% reduction in the LV end-systolic volume from time of implant to 6 months.

Results: Out of total patients in the cohort, 68% were men. Mean age of the patients was 65 ± 11 years, and left ventricular ejection fraction (LVEF) was 28 ± 8%. Longer RV-LV durations were found to be significantly associated with CRT response (p <0.01) for all the patients of cohort. Furthermore, there was an increase in benefit of AVO with prolongation in RV-LV duration. At the longest quartile, there was a 4.26 × greater odds of a remodeling response in comparison to nominal atrioventricular delays (p = 0.010).

Conclusion: Interventricular delay at baseline predicted the CRT response. At long RV-LV durations, AVO can result in increased possibility of reverse remodeling with CRT. AVO and LV lead location which were optimized to maximize interventricular delay may work synergistically for increasing CRT response.

COMMENT

Atrioventricular optimization (AVO) trial. Patients with prolonged right ventricular (RV) to left ventricular (LV) time were also more likely to benefit from atrioventricular

*Redrafted abstract

delay optimization. Thus, combining LV pacing at a site with maximal activation delay with subsequent AVO may have additional benefit.

Prolonged interventricular delay, as measured by the difference in activation time between the RV and LV leads, is associated with better cardiac resynchronization therapy (CRT) response. The present study was designed to assess whether AVO further improves the benefit of pacing at long RV-LV durations. A simple measure of interventricular delay was used, that is, the time between RV and LV electrograms at the sites of final lead implantation, and found significant correlation with CRT response in the SmartDelay.

This study brings out two important messages:

1. Atrioventricular optimization, using an algorithm that promotes fusions with intrinsic conduction and maximizes acute hemodynamic response (SmartDelay), is associated with improved CRT response compared with nominal AV delay programming when pacing at sites with long RV-LV durations. There is no benefit of AVO at pacing sites with short RV-LV durations.

2. The CRT nonresponder rate can be decreased significantly by choosing pacing sites or pacing electrodes of multipolar leads with long RV-LV duration (>70 ms) and using AVO.

ARTICLE 5

Electrocardiographic Features Differentiating Arrhythmogenic Right Ventricular Cardiomyopathy from an Athlete's Heart

Brosnan MJ, Te Riele ASJM, Bosman LP, et al. Electrocardiographic features differentiating arrhythmogenic right ventricular cardiomyopathy from an athlete's heart.
JACC Clin Electrophysiol. 2018;4(12):1613-25.

*Abstract**

Anterior T-wave inversion (TWI) [TWI in leads V1 to V4 (TWI_{V1-V4})] is a greatest area of ambiguity in interpretation of electrocardiogram (ECG) in athletes. It is because it is common in both the healthy athletes and athletes with arrhythmogenic right ventricular cardiomyopathy (ARVC). So, ECG evaluation is being added into athletes' preparticipation screening with rising frequency. Precordial TWI is prevalent in both the athletes with ARVC and endurance athletes. In ECG interpretation, this diagnostic overlap is still a limitation.

*Redrafted abstract

In this study, total 200 subjects with TWI_{V1-V4} were included. Out of these, 100 were healthy athletes and 100 were ARVC patients matched 1:1 for age, sex, and ethnicity (age 21 ± 5 years for athletes vs. 22 ± 5 years for ARVC patients; 47% male; 97% Caucasian). Presence of J point Elevation (JPE), TWI, left ventricular hypertrophy (LVH), and premature ventricular contractions (PVCs) was evaluated. The study indicated that JPE prevalence is affected by age, gender, and ethnicity. It is not adequately specific finding that is helpful in athletes' ECG screening. Contrary to this, spontaneous PVCs, low QRS voltages, and TWI were found to be more strongly associated with ARVC. It can be argued that the lack of these novel markers was of adequately robust negative predictive value to be beneficial in screening. Presently, the latter two of these three markers are not included in the criteria for differentiating between the heart and pathology in athletes.

COMMENT

One of the greatest areas of ambiguity in the interpretation of electrocardiograms (ECGs) in athletes is anterior T-wave inversion (TWI) [TWI in leads V1 to V4 (TWI_{V1-V4})] because it is common in both arrhythmogenic right ventricular cardiomyopathy (ARVC) and healthy athletes. ECG evaluation is being incorporated into preparticipation screening of athletes with increasing frequency. Precordial TWI is prevalent in both endurance athletes and those with ARVC, and this diagnostic overlap continues to be one of the limitations in ECG interpretation.

This study examined 200 subjects with TWI $_{V1-V4}$, including 100 healthy athletes and 100 ARVC patients matched 1:1 for age, sex, and ethnicity (age: 21 ± 5 years for athletes vs. 22 ± 5 years for ARVC patients; 47% male; 97% Caucasian). The presence of TWI, J point Elevation (JPE), premature ventricular contractions (PVCs), and left ventricular hypertrophy (LVH) were assessed.

The results suggested that prevalence of JPE is influenced by age, sex, and ethnicity, and is not an adequately specific finding to be useful in ECG screening of athletes. In contrast, TWI, spontaneous PVCs, and low QRS voltages were more strongly associated with ARVC, and it could be argued that the absence of these novel markers was of sufficiently robust negative predictive value to be useful for screening. The latter two of these three markers are not currently considered in criteria to differentiate between the heart and pathology in athletes.

ARTICLE 6

Outcomes of Catheter Ablation of Ventricular Tachycardia Based on Etiology in Nonischemic Heart Disease: An International Ventricular Tachycardia Ablation Center Collaborative Study

Vaseghi M, Hu TY, Tung R, et al. Outcomes of catheter ablation of ventricular tachycardia based on etiology in nonischemic heart disease: An international ventricular tachycardia ablation center collaborative study. *JACC Clin Electrophysiol. 2018;4(9):1141-50.)*

*Abstract**

Background and Objectives: In patients with nonischemic cardiomyopathy (NICM), the outcomes of catheter ablation of ventricular tachycardia (VT) may be associated with etiology of NICM. This study was aimed at characterizing the outcomes of VT ablation across the NICM etiologies and adjusting these outcomes by patient-related comorbidities, which can explain differences in arrhythmia recurrence rates.

Methods: In this study, data from 2,075 patients, who have structural heart disease and referred for catheter ablation of VT from 12 international centers, was retrospectively analyzed. Characteristics of patients and outcomes were recorded for six most common NICM etiologies. To adjust for potential confounders, multivariable cox proportional hazards modeling was used.

Results: There were total 780 NICM patients. Mean age of the patients was 57 ± 14 years; 18% were women. Left ventricular ejection fraction was noted to be 37 ± 13%. Out of 780 NICM patients, for dilated idiopathic cardiomyopathy (DICM) underlying prevalence was 66%; for arrhythmogenic right ventricular cardiomyopathy (ARVC)—13%; for valvular cardiomyopathy—6%; for myocarditis—6%; for hypertrophic cardiomyopathy—4%; and for sarcoidosis—3%. 1 year freedom from VT was found to be 69%; freedom from VT, heart transplantation, and death was observed to be 62%. In unadjusted competing risk analysis, VT ablation in ARVC showed superior VT-free survival (82%) in comparison to DICM (p ≤0.01). Valvular cardiomyopathy was noted to be having poorest unadjusted VT-free survival (47%) (p <0.01). After adjusting for comorbidities (which include age, ejection fraction, heart failure severity, prior ablation, and antiarrhythmic medication use), myocarditis, ARVC, and DICM showed comparable outcomes, while valvular cardiomyopathy, sarcoidosis, and hypertrophic cardiomyopathy demonstrated highest risk of VT recurrence.

Conclusion: Catheter ablation of VT in NICM is effective. In patients with NICM, etiology is a significant predictor of outcomes, with myocarditis, DICM, and ARVC having comparable but superior outcomes to valvular cardiomyopathy, sarcoidosis, and hypertrophic cardiomyopathy, after adjusting for the potential covariates.

*Redrafted abstract

COMMENT

Catheter ablation for VT in NICM has shown to have lower success rates and recurrences compared with ischemic cardiomyopathy in previous studies.

ARTICLE 7

Risk Models for Prediction of Implantable Cardioverter-defibrillator Benefit: Insights from the DANISH Trial

Kristensen SL, Levy WC, Shadman R, et al. Risk models for prediction of implantable cardioverter-defibrillator benefit: Insights from the DANISH trial.
JACC Heart Fail. 2019;7(8):717-24.

*Abstract**

For primary prevention, the use of an implantable cardioverter-defibrillator (ICD) is recommended in patients with heart failure (HF) and reduced ejection fraction regardless of etiology.

However, the results of Danish study to Assess the Efficacy of ICDs in Patients with Nonischemic Systolic Heart Failure on mortality (DANISH) trial created some doubts to the benefits of ICD in nonischemic cardiomyopathy particularly in older patients.

Combinations of previously validated HF risk prediction models were applied in this study for identification of patients who had nonischemic HF with a greater risk of sudden cardiac death (SCD), both absolutely and relatively, who would be more likely to get benefit from an ICD. In patients enrolled in the DANISH trial, the Seattle Proportional Risk Model (SPRM) (estimates the proportional risk of sudden vs. nonsudden death) and the Seattle Heart Failure Model (SHFM) (estimates overall mortality) were used.

With the following parameters, the SPRM score predicts the likelihood of SCD versus nonsudden death:

- Increasing relative likelihood of SCD: Younger age, male sex, higher body mass index, New York Heart Association (NYHA) functional class II versus NYHA functional class III/IV, low left ventricular ejection fraction (LVEF), and use of digoxin.
- Conversely, hyper/hypotension, diabetes, hyponatremia, and renal dysfunction decrease relative SCD likelihood as estimated by the SPRM.

All-cause mortality is predicted by SHFM with following parameters associated with:

- An increased risk: older age, male sex, reduced LVEF, higher NYHA functional class, hyponatremia, ischemic etiology, uric acid, and high/low hemoglobin,
- Lower risk is associated with high cholesterol or lymphocytes, high systolic blood pressure, use of beta blockers, statins, mineralocorticoid receptor antagonists, and having an cardiac resynchronization therapy (CRT) or ICD.

*Redrafted abstract

Results: In patients having SPRM score above the median (n = 558), ICD implantation decreased all-cause mortality [hazard ratio (HR), 0.63, 95% confidence interval (CI) 0.43–0.94), while patients with lower SPRM scores (n = 558) had no effect (HR 1.08, 95% CI 0.78–1.49, p for interaction = 0.04).

Conclusion: In patients with nonischemic systolic HF, the advantage of implanting an ICD for primary prevention of SCD has been questioned because of improved pharmacological treatment. This analysis suggests that risk prediction models can provide guidance for identification of patients who are more likely to benefit from an ICD. Implantation of an ICD decreases the risk of SCD by nearly 50% among patients who have nonischemic systolic HF, regardless of predicted risk.

Further knowledge is required in this field before applying this knowledge in clinical practice, specifically in terms of understanding the pathophysiologic mechanisms that result in refractory malignant arrhythmia. Till then guideline-based therapy will hold the key.

ARTICLE 8

Ventricular Arrhythmias and Sudden Cardiac Arrest in Takotsubo Cardiomyopathy: Incidence, Predictive Factors, and Clinical Implications

Jesel L, Berthon C, Messas N, et al. Ventricular arrhythmias and sudden cardiac arrest in Takotsubo cardiomyopathy: Incidence, predictive factors, and clinical implications.
Heart Rhythm. 2018;15:1171-8.

*Abstract**

Background: Takotsubo cardiomyopathy (TTC) is a transient cardiomyopathy related with stress. There may be occurrence of life-threatening arrhythmias (LTA) which can worsen the prognosis.

Objective: This study was aimed at assessing the incidence and outcome of LTA in TTC, along with the predictive factors and clinical implications.

Methods: Total 214 consecutive cases of TTC were studied over 8 years. Entire cohort was divided into two groups—patients with LTA (LTA group) and those patients without (non-LTA group). LTA was defined as ventricular fibrillation, ventricular tachycardia, or cardiac arrest.

Results: In 10.7% (n = 23) of patients, LTA occurred mainly in the first 24 hours of hospitalization— cardiac arrest (n = 10; 5 asystole, 3 complete heart block, and 2 sinoatrial block), ventricular

---

*Redrafted abstract

fibrillation (n = 11), and ventricular tachycardia (n = 2). LTAs were found to be associated with lower left ventricular ejection fraction (LVEF) and high rate of the conduction disturbances. There was a significant increase in the LTA group in in-hospital (39.1% vs. 8.9%, p <0.001) and 1-year mortality (47.8% vs. 14.1%, p <0.001) rates. Independent predictors of LTA were LVEF and QRS duration more than 105 ms. In cases with implanted device, conduction disturbances remained after the index event in spite of complete recovery of LVEF. During follow-up, there was no ventricular arrhythmia (VA) recurrence.

Conclusion: Life-threatening arrhythmias occur early among patients who present with TTC; LTAs are found to be associated with significantly worse short-term and long-term prognosis. Independent predictors of LTA are left ventricular impairment and QRS duration more than 105 ms.

Ventricular arrhythmias took place in the acute phase without further recurrence noted among hospital survivors, while severe conduction disorders remained during long-term follow-up. These results can have implications on the choice of device therapy for this particular patient subgroup.

COMMENT

Takotsubo cardiomyopathy (TTC), a stress-related reversible cardiomyopathy, is characterized by transient left ventricular dysfunction with wall motion abnormalities which are global and occur in the absence of hemodynamically significant coronary obstruction. In most cases, the prognosis is favorable with recovery of LVEF within several days. During acute phase, these patients are prone to LTA and this generally has a poor prognosis. In the present study, 214 consecutive cases of TTC were examined over a period of 8 years. LTAs occurred in 10.7% of patients. LTAs were associated with lower LVEF and a high rate of conduction disturbances. In TTC cases complicated by LTA, hospital stay was longer and in-hospital,

cardiovascular, and 1-year mortality rates were dramatically increased. LVEF and QRS duration >105 ms were independent predictors of LTA onset. In cases of device implantation, conduction disturbances persisted after the index event despite complete recovery of LVEF whereas no ventricular arrhythmia (VA) recurrence was noted during follow-up.

In this study, the prognostic implication of LTA was severe LTA onset dramatically affected short- and long-term mortality. Notably, patients presenting with LTA who survived to hospital discharge have a favorable prognosis, with none of them encountering cardiovascular death or an arrhythmic event during the 1st year of follow-up.

Section 9

Left Ventricular Assist Device and Transplant

Section Editor: Thirugnanasambandan Sunder

Predicted Heart Mass is the Optimal Metric for Size Match in Heart Transplantation

Kransdorf EP, Kittleson MM, Benck LR, et al. Predicted heart mass is the optimal metric for size match in heart transplantation.
J Heart Lung Transplant. 2019;38(2):156-65.

Abstract*

Background: Traditionally, donor-recipient size match is evaluated by body weight. This study is aimed at evaluating ability of five size match metrics, predicted heart mass (PHM), weight, height, body mass index (BMI) and body surface area (BSA), for predicting 1-year mortality after heart transplant. Another aim of the study was to evaluate the impact of size match on donor heart turn down for size.

Methods: The study cohort included 19,168 adult heart transplant recipients in the United Network for Organ Sharing registry from 2007 to 2016. Using the donor-recipient ratio for each metric, each size match metric was divided into seven groups of equal size. Single and multivariable Cox proportional hazard models were constructed for mortality 1-year after transplant.

Results: Recipients in the severely (donor-recipient PHM ratio, 0.54–0.86) undersized group for PHM had increase in mortality, with hazard ratio of 1.34 [95% confidence interval (CI), 1.13–1.59, p <0.001]. No increased risk of death at 1-year was observed if donors were undersized for height, weight, BMI, or BSA. It was observed that 32% of heart offers turned down for donor size would be acceptable by using a PHM threshold of ≥0.86 and that 14% of heart offers accepted (majority of which are female donor to male recipient) were less than this threshold.

Conclusion: To predict mortality after heart transplant, PHM is considered as the optimal donor-recipient size match metric for predicting mortality. Most of the offers turned down for donor size were more than the threshold for adequacy of size match by PHM identified. Therefore, the use of PHM can improve utilization of donor heart and post-transplant survival.

*Redrafted abstract

COMMENT

Heart transplantation (HT) remains the gold standard for treatment of end-stage heart failure in eligible patients. There are an estimated 26 million people with heart failure worldwide. Annually about 5500 heart transplants are being done worldwide. Hence there are much more patients waiting for heart transplant—who could deteriorate and may not survive till an organ is available.

In India, HT is now increasingly performed in many states of the country with good results. While the accurate burden of patients with end-stage heart failure in India is not available, the number of patients is certainly large and exceeds the number of usable donor hearts available. Given the scarce resource, steps must be taken to ensure that the donor heart is used appropriately so that the outcomes are best, and the precious organ is not wasted in a mortality which can be predicted and prevented.

Size matching is one of the important parameters, among many others, which the transplant clinician considers while accepting or declining an organ. Traditionally, the body weight has been used as a measure of heart size and the guidelines by International Society of Heart and Lung Transplantation (ISHLT) suggest accepting a heart from donors within 30% of recipient body weight and within 20% of recipient body weight if the donor is a female. Body weight does not always correlate to heart size. Other parameters such as height, body mass index (BMI), body surface area (BSA) have also been used by many centers with respect to size matching. Predicted heart mass (PHM) has been calculated using formula incorporating age, sex, height and weight.

In this article, the authors have looked at 659,231 heart offers—out of which 19,772 hearts were accepted and 631,517 hearts were declined. They have used five metrics—body weight, height, BMI, BSA and PHM and classed patients into seven groups based on donor-recipient ratio for each metric—severely undersized (U3), moderately under-sized (U2), mildly undersized (U1), well matched (septile 4), mildly oversized (O1), moderately oversized (O2) and severely oversized (O3) and compared the early and 1-year mortality in these groups.

While there were no survival differences between the seven groups when weight, height, BMI and BSA were used, there was significant difference when PHM was used—particularly in the severely undersized group (U3). In this group, the donor-recipient ratio was (0.543–0.863) with 1-month mortality of 41% and 5-month mortality of 68%. Furthermore, recipients in the U3 group experienced increased mortality with hazard ratio of 1.34 (95% CI 1.13–1.59, p <0.001). The authors point out that when the donor-recipient ratio using PHM is greater than 0.85, there is no increase in mortality. Using 0.85 PHM ratio as a threshold, they found that 30,332 hearts which were declined based on size/weight could have been used with no increase in mortality.

The authors conclude that PHM is the optimal metric for size matching and that using this would allow more hearts to be used. Dr Michael Givertz, in his editorial in the same issue, suggests that "the use of hearts from donors whose PHM is at least 0.86 that of the recipient is uniformly safe". Alternatively, he adds, "one could state that donor organs with a PHM >10% to 15% below that of the recipient is not recommended".

In our country, body weight is used more often for size matching which assumes a direct correlation between body weight and heart size. It appears logical to assume that using body weight alone as a surrogate for heart size may be inaccurate and using a model which incorporates age, sex, height and weight may be more appropriate.

Further data analysis in Indian patients would help make recommendations in our scenario.

While it is a little cumbersome to compute PHM, its usage would ensure better size matching and increase donor pool.

ARTICLE 2

Donor Predicted Heart Mass as Predictor of Primary Graft Dysfunction

Gong TA, Joseph SM, Lima B, et al. Donor predicted heart mass as predictor of primary graft dysfunction. *J Heart Lung Transplant. 2018;37:826-35.*

Abstract*

Background: Concern about the hazards related with undersized donor hearts has hindered the use of otherwise viable allografts for transplantation. It is reported by previous studies that predicted heart mass (PHM) can provide better size matching in cardiac transplantation as compared to total body weight (TBW). This study was aimed at evaluating whether size-matching donor hearts by PHM is a better predictor of primary graft dysfunction (PGD) as compared to matching by TBW.

Methods: Records of consecutive adult cardiac transplants conducted in a single academic hospital between 2012 and 2016 have been evaluated. Patients implanted with hearts undersized by 30% or more were compared to those implanted with donor hearts matched for size (within 30%); analysis was performed both for undersizing by PHM and for undersizing by TBW. Primary outcome considered in study was moderate/severe PGD within 24 hours, as per 2014 International Society for Heart and Lung Transplantation consensus. One-year survival was the secondary outcome.

Results: Out of 253 patients, 12% (n = 30) and 8% (n = 21) received hearts undersized by PHM and TBW, respectively. Overall rate of moderate/severe PGD was found to be 13% (33 patients). PGD was observed to be associated with undersizing—if performed by PHM (p = 0.007), but not if performed by TBW (p = 0.49).

*Redrafted abstract

There was no difference in 1-year survival between groups (log-rank, p >0.8). It was confirmed by multivariate analysis that undersizing donor hearts by PHM, but not by TBW, was predictive of the moderate/severe PGD [odds ratio (OR) 3.3, 95% confidence interval (CI) 1.3–8.6].

Conclusion: Undersized donor hearts by 30% or more by PHM may enhance rates of PGD after transplantation, which confirms that PHM gives more clinically appropriate size matching as compared to TBW. Better size matching may finally allow for expansion of the donor pool.

COMMENT

Primary graft dysfunction (PGD) after heart transplantation (HT)—without a clear precipitating cause—refers to significant decrease in systolic function of donor left ventricle (LV), right ventricle (RV) or both occurring within 24 hours of heart transplantation with hemodynamic compromise requiring multiple inotropes or mechanical circulatory support—and which is not due to rejection, fluid overload or recipient pulmonary hypertension.

Primary graft dysfunction is the leading cause of death and accounts for up to 40% of early deaths occurring within 1-month of HT. The reported incidence ranges from 1% to 31%.

The International Society of Heart and Lung Transplantation (ISHLT) released a consensus document in 2014 about clear definition and grading of PGD following HT. The exact etiology of PGD remains elusive and it is believed to be multifactorial with donor, recipient and procedural factors playing a role. Scoring systems predicting development of PGD have been described. RADIAL score has six risk factors such as— Right atrial pressure >10 mm Hg, recipient age >60 years, Diabetes mellitus, Inotrope dependence, donor age >30 years, Length of ischemic time >240 minutes. Each factor

has a score of 1 and the sum of all forms the RADIAL score. Higher the score—greater the likelihood of PGD.

In this study, the authors used size matching by predicted heart mass (PHM) and total body weight (TBW) and looked at development of moderate/severe PGD as primary endpoint. Secondary endpoints included hospital mortality, intensive care unit (ICU) and hospital stay, rejection, infection, blood products used. The comparison was between recipients with undersized hearts (>30% undersizing) and those with "normal sized" hearts (<30% undersizing). Undersizing was computed using PHM and TBW. There was a marked increase in PGD when undersizing by PHM >30%. There was no such increase while using TBW to size-match.

It appears that size matching by TBW alone may not be accurate. Using PHM would serve to increase donor pool by allowing usage of organs which may be turned down based on body weight alone.

Clearly this is a single center experience and one would agree that further analysis in larger multicenter cohorts would be needed. By avoiding severe undersizing (>30%) by PHM, the transplant clinicians would be able to choose the correct donor for a given recipient.

*Redrafted abstract

ARTICLE 3

Validation of the International Society for Heart and Lung Transplantation Primary Graft Dysfunction Instrument in Heart Transplantation

Foroutan F, Alba AC, Stein M, et al. Validation of the International Society for Heart and Lung Transplantation primary graft dysfunction instrument in heart transplantation.
J Heart Lung Transplant. 2019;38(3):260-6.

*Abstract**

Background: The International Society for Heart and Lung Transplantation (ISHLT), in 2014, developed classification instrument for left ventricular (LV) and isolated right ventricular (RV) primary graft dysfunction (PGD) postheart transplant. LV-PGD is classified by this instrument as mild, moderate, or severe. Predictive validity of this instrument is evaluated in this study.

Methods: This is a cohort study including 412 consecutive patients who were transplanted at the Toronto General Hospital and Ottawa Heart Institute (Canada) between 2004 and 2015. By using the ISHLT instrument, LV-PGD was classified as mild, moderate, or severe. For evaluating predictive validity, the association between LV-PGD severity and 1-year post-transplant mortality was assessed by using a Cox regression model adjusted for recipient age.

Results: Cohort included predominantly male (71%) patients. Mean age of the patients was 50 ± 13 years; mean donor age was 38 ± 14 years, with 25% being female donors. Mean ischemic time was 3.7 ± 1.1 hours. LV-PGD was severe in 3.9% patients, moderate in 9.5%, and mild in 3.6%. All levels of LV-PGD were observed to be associated with increase in 1-year mortality, with a gradient in the association between mild, moderate, and severe. A statistically significant association was observed for moderate LV-PGD and severe LV-PGD [mild: hazard ratio (HR) 2.4, 95% confidence interval (CI) 0.6–10.2; moderate: HR 7.0, 95% CI 3.4–14.6; severe: HR 15.9, 95% CI 7.2–35.0].

Conclusion: The ISHLT LV-PGD classification convincingly recognizes substantial increased risk of death at 1-year. An increase in gradient of risk was also noted among patients who had moderate or severe LV-PGD.

COMMENT

Primary graft dysfunction (PGD) after heart transplantation (HT) refers to impaired heart function without any clear precipitating cause—unlike secondary dysfunction

*Redrafted abstract

which may be due to rejection, irreversible pulmonary hypertension or fluid overload. It refers to significant impairment of systolic function of left ventricle (LV), right ventricle (RV) or both within 24 hours of HT with hemodynamic compromise requiring multiple inotropes or mechanical circulatory support.

There were different criteria used to diagnose PGD after HT and the incidence of PGD has ranged between 1% and 31% based on the definitions or criteria used. Wide variability in diagnosing PGD led to wide ranging incidence with difficulties in prognosticating these patients and developing appropriate management protocols.

While PGD following lung transplantation has been addressed much earlier in 2005 by a working group of the International Society for Heart and Lung Transplantation (ISHLT), it was not until 2014 that guidelines were issued by the ISHLT which clearly defines and classifies PGD after HT. The ISHLT defines "PGD after HT as graft dysfunction, not due to rejection, fluid overload or pulmonary hypertension, which occurs within 24 hours of HT".

The ISHLT classified the severity of PGD as LV-PGD, biventricular (BV)-PGD or RV-PGD.

Based on the level of support required LV-PGD and BV-PGD were further classified into mild, moderate or severe.

Using the PGD instrument issued by ISHLT, there were a few studies reported 30-day mortality following HT ranging from 31% to 50% due to severe PGD. However, data about 1-year mortality based on severity was lacking. The RADIAL score is a risk predicting score which predicts early PGD—but does not stratify severity of PGD.

In this study, the authors have looked at the clinical course of 412 heart transplant recipients for a 11-year period from 2004 until 2015 and have evaluated the predictive validity of the ISHLT PGD classification. They point out that this is the first study to validate the ISHLT PGD classification at 1-year, and found that 1-year mortality correlates well with the severity of PGD—with heightened mortality for patients with moderate/severe PGD.

This study had 100% follow-up at 1-year and validates the ISHLT classification. Further studies are needed which—in addition to identifying PGD (e.g. RADIAL score)—will help to predict the severity of PGD post-HT. Such data will help the clinician in proper selection of recipients for a given organ with improved outcomes.

ARTICLE 4

Risk of Severe Primary Graft Dysfunction in Patients Bridged to Heart Transplantation with Continuous-flow Left Ventricular Assist Devices

Truby LK, Takeda K, Topkara VK, et al. Risk of severe primary graft dysfunction in patients bridged to heart transplantation with continuous-flow left ventricular assist devices.
J Heart Lung Transplant. 2018;37(12):1433-42.

Abstract*

Background: Primary graft dysfunction (PGD) is still an important cause of post-transplant morbidity and mortality. In the contemporary era, exact mechanism and risk factors for this phenomenon are still not known.

Methods: In this study, we reviewed adult patients who underwent heart transplantation (HT) between 2009 and 2017 at our institution. Severe PGD was defined in study as requirement for mechanical circulatory support (MCS) within the first 24 hours following HT. For identifying risk factors for severe PGD, multivariate logistic regression analysis was used, focusing on patients bridged to transplant (BTT) with continuous-flow left ventricular assist device (CF-LVAD).

Results: Severe PGD was present in 11.7% (56 of 480) HT patients. Among severe PGD patients, 80% were BTT with a CF-LVAD [odds ratio (OR), 3.86, 95% confidence interval (CI), 1.94–7.68, p <0.001]. In BTT patients, significant associations were identified between more than 1-year of CF-LVAD support (OR 2.48, 95% CI 1.14–5.40, p = 0.022), pre-HT creatinine (OR 3.35, 95% CI 1.42–7.92, p = 0.006), elevated central venous pressure/pulmonary capillary wedge pressure (CVP/PCWP) ratio (OR 3.32, 95% CI 1.04–10.60, p = 0.043); use of amiodarone before HT (OR 2.69, 95% CI 1.20–6.20, p = 0.022); and severe PGD. In this contemporary cohort, RADIAL score did not accurately predict severe PGD. Patients who developed severe PGD had reduced 1-year post-transplant survival (78.3% vs. 91.8%, p = 0.007).

Conclusion: CF-LVAD use as BTT is found to be associated with an increase in risk of severe PGD. Increase in time on device support, right ventricular dysfunction, renal dysfunction as evaluated by CVP/PCWP ratio, and pretransplant amiodarone may recognize high-risk patients. Future research that focuses on optimal timing of device implantation and transplantation along with underlying mechanisms of PGD are required.

COMMENT

Left ventricular assist devices (LVADs) are mechanical devices which assist the diseased left ventricle in pumping blood from the left ventricle on to the aorta. The first successful LAVD implant was done in 1966 by Dr Michael DeBakey where in a paracorporeal (external) circuit was used. These devices were initially large and with technological advances miniaturizing was possible to allow fully implantable devices inside the patient's chest with a drive line connected to an external, portable and rechargeable power source. The first-generation LVADs had pulsatile flow and then subsequently continuous flow pumps were developed.

These long-term, durable mechanical devices were initially developed to provide support as a bridged to transplant (BTT) but have subsequently also been used as a bridge to recovery or in some instances as

*Redrafted abstract

a destination therapy (DT). The needs for anticoagulation with its attendant bleeding complications, infective complications of the drive line, pump thrombosis with embolic risk are the main complications.

Short-term percutaneously implantable LVADs have also been developed which has a role predominantly in patients with cardiogenic shock and who need support for a few hours to few days.

The majority of LVADs are implanted as BTT. The current generations of LVADs use continuous flow pumps and are indicated in patients with end-stage heart failure (HF) who are deteriorating while on the waiting list for heart transplantation (HT). They are very beneficial in that they preserve the function of other organs like liver and kidney and prevent development of irreversible pulmonary hypertension. By virtue of the above effects, they decrease the mortality of patients on the waiting list for HT. In patient not eligible for HT, they provide good quality of life when used as DT. The risk of bleeding, thromboembolism, stroke and infection needs to be balanced with its benefits in preventing multiorgan failure and reducing mortality while awaiting HT.

In this article, the authors have analyzed the risk of severe primary graft dysfunction (PGD) following HT in patients who were bridged with continuous flow (CF) LVAD. They have defined severe PGD as the need for mechanical circulatory support (MCS) within the first 24 hours after HT. Among 480 HT recipients, 56 patients developed severe PGD. Eighty percent of severe PGD were in patients with BTT using CF-LVAD.

Hence, they further analyzed the cohort of 263 patients who were BTT using CF-LVAD and identified the following pre-HT risk factors for developing severe PGD in patients with CF-LVAD.

The risk factors for developing severe PGD include duration of CF-LVAD greater than 1-year, elevated pre-HT creatinine, elevated central venous pressure (CVP)/pulmonary capillary wedge pressure (PCWP) ratio and pre-HT use of amiodarone.

The paradox to contend with by the transplant physician—is the role of CF-LVAD in decreasing waiting list mortality while increasing the risk of severe PGD after HT. It has been suggested that prolonged support with CF-LVAD may cause negative remodeling of the vasculature with increased post-HT morbidity and mortality. Attempting to reduce the duration on CF-LVAD support by timing device implant more appropriately needs further studies—because timing of device explant and HT can never be predicted—and the time on CF-LVAD support is a "nonmodifiable" risk factor—at this point in time.

Better medical management and maintaining optimal fluid balance to aim for low CVP/PCWP ratio and avoidance of amiodarone pre-HT while on CF-LVAD would help in reducing severe PGD and improve HT outcomes.

In India, LVAD is not frequently implanted mainly because it is very expensive and patients have to fund for the device themselves. In such scenarios, it is even more important to consider reducing all possible risk factors which can contribute to severe PGD.

ARTICLE 5

Left Ventricular Assist Devices versus Medical Management in Ambulatory Heart Failure Patients: An Analysis of INTERMACS Profiles 4 and 5 to 7 from the ROADMAP Study

Shah KB, Starling RC, Rogers JG, et al. Left ventricular assist devices versus medical management in ambulatory heart failure patients: An analysis of INTERMACS Profiles 4 and 5 to 7 from the ROADMAP study.
J Heart Lung Transplant. 2018;37(6):706-14.

*Abstract**

Background: The ROADMAP (Risk Assessment and Comparative Effectiveness of Left Ventricular Assist Device and Medical Management in Ambulatory Heart Failure Patients) study demonstrated that survival with improved functional status was better with left ventricular assist device (LVAD) therapy in comparison with optimal medical management (OMM) among ambulatory, noninotrope-dependent [INTERMACS (IM) Profiles 4 to 7] patients. For studying more balanced cohorts and better define which patients can benefit from LVAD implantation, patients enrolled in ROADMAP were re-evaluated when stratified by INTERMACS profile (Profile 4 and Profiles 5 to 7).

Methods: The primary endpoint was survival on original therapy with improvement in 6-minute walk distance 75 meters or more at 1-year. The primary endpoint, adverse events (AEs), actuarial survival, and health-related quality of life (HRQOL) were assessed.

Results: For INTERMACS Profile 4 (IM4), more number of LVAD patients met the primary endpoint in comparison with OMM patients [40% vs. 15%; odds ratio 3.9 (1.2–12.7), p = 0.024]. However, no statistically significant difference was observed for INTERMACS Profiles IM 5 to 7 (IM5-7).

The event-free survival on original therapy at 2 years was more for LVAD as compared to that for OMM patients in both IM4 (67% vs. 28%; p <0.001) and IM5-7 (76% vs. 49%; p = 0.025) profile groups. Composite endpoints of survival on original therapy with improved HRQOL or depression were found to be better with LVAD as compared to OMM in IM4, but not in IM5-7. AEs trended higher in LVAD in comparison with OMM patients in both profile groups. Rates of rehospitalization for LVAD versus OMM were comparable between treatment arms in IM4 (82% vs. 86%; p = 0.780), but were found to be greater for LVAD in IM5-7 (93% vs. 71%; p = 0.016).

Conclusion: LVAD patients in IM4, but not in IM5-7, are more likely to meet the primary endpoint and have improved HRQOL and depression in comparison with OMM, even with AEs usually being more frequent. LVAD therapy along with current technology may be useful in select IM4 patients, but it can be deferred for majority of the IM5-7 patients who should be followed closely because of the high frequency of failure of treatment.

**Redrafted abstract

COMMENT

The ROADMAP study was a prospective, non-randomized, multicentric (n = 41), controlled, observational study to evaluate effectiveness of optimal medical management (OMM) and left ventricular assist device (LVAD) in ambulatory heart failure (HF) patients (NYHA III/IV) who were followed up for 2 years. The results of the study were published in 2017 which showed that LVADs were superior to OMM in terms of survival and improved physical performance, however, with an increase in adverse events (AEs).

Left ventricular assist devices have been shown to be beneficial in patients with end-stage HF and are best used as a bridged to transplant (BTT) with preservation of end-organ functions. However, the risk of AE—mainly bleeding and thrombosis when affecting the central nervous system (CNS) and causing stroke can be devastating. Furthermore, the longer the time on LVAD support, higher is the risk of severe primary graft dysfunction (PGD) post-HT. Dr Christopher Hayward, in his editorial, points out that "Late referral, however, is often not because of lack of knowledge on the referrers' part about hemodynamic benefit of mechanical circulatory support (MCS), but because of concern about AEs".

To time the implantation of LVAD is crucial and can also be challenging. While it confers hemodynamic benefits with preservation of end-organ function, the adverse effects can be significant. The treating physician needs to balance the risk of LVAD-associated AEs with risks of worsening HF on OMM.

In this study, the authors have gone deeper to analyze the RAODMAP cohort and re-evaluated ROADMAP ambulatory HF patients based on INTERMACS (Interagency Registry for Mechanically Assisted Circulatory Support) profiles. Two groups—INTERMACS 4 (IM4) and INTERMACS 5-7 (IM5-7) were formed and outcomes compared at the end of 2 years. In the RAODMAP cohort, IM4 patients were the most symptomatic, while IM5-7 were the least sick of patients.

At 2 years, LVADs in IM4 patients were more likely to meet primary composite endpoint of survival with improved 6-minute walk distance >75 meters, and reported better quality of life than OMM, despite the AEs. The authors, therefore, conclude that LVADs have a role in selected HF patients in IM4 level.

As pointed out by Dr Christopher Hayward in his editorial, significant advances have been made both in LVAD technology and OMM (valsartan-sacubitril) after the results of ROADMAP study and therefore balance each other. Timing is of paramount importance while advising LVAD implant. He adds that further developments with reduction in AEs will be needed before LVADs can be recommended to the broader HF population.

The eighth annual INTERMACS report (2017) with a special focus on AE, demonstrate only minimal advantage of LVADs in patients with ambulatory HF due to major AEs and may be beneficial in a select group of patients.

For our patients, given that LVADs are expensive and costs must be borne by the patients—caution must be exercised in deciding the right time for implanting LVADs so that most of the benefits of LVADs can be harnessed, while keeping AEs to a minimum.

ARTICLE 6

Risk of Stroke Early after Implantation of a Left Ventricular Assist Device

Samura T, Yoshioka D, Toda K, et al. Risk of stroke early after implantation of a left ventricular assist device. *J Thorac Cardiovasc Surg. 2019;157(1):259-67.*

*Abstract**

Objectives: Stroke is one of the major adverse events after left ventricular assist device implantation. Risk of stroke is the highest immediately after left ventricular assist device implantation and then increases again in chronic periods. There is no study that has analyzed risk factors for stroke in acute phase. We investigated the risk factors for stroke in the acute phase after left ventricular assist device implantation in the present study.

Methods: Between October, 2005 and December, 2016, 158 consecutive patients (mean age, 43 ± 14 years; 34% were women) underwent continuous-flow left ventricular assist device [50 HeartMate II (Abbott Medical, Abbott Park, Ill), 38 DuraHeart (Terumo Heart, Ann Arbor, Mich), 33 Jarvik2000 (Jarvik Heart, New York, NY), 23 EVAHEART (Sun Medical, Moriyama City, Japan), 14 HeartWare (Framingham, Mass)] implantation in our institution. We analyzed the risk factors for a symptomatic stroke within 90 days after left ventricular assist device implantation.

Results: Stroke occurred in 28 patients in the acute phase after left ventricular assist device implantation. Multivariate analysis revealed that low cardiac output [odds ratio 0.25 (0.07–0.92), p = 0.024] during postoperative 12–24 hours was the only independent risk factor for stroke in the acute phase. Patients with stroke in the acute phase had higher serum lactate dehydrogenase levels at any point until postoperative 14 days. Patients with the HeartMate II device particularly showed a statistically significant negative relationship between cardiac output during postoperative 12–24 hours and serum lactate dehydrogenase levels at postoperative 14 days (r = −0.313, p = 0.03).

Conclusion: Our study demonstrated that patients with perioperative lower cardiac output and higher lactate dehydrogenase level developed stroke in the acute phase after left ventricular assist device implantation. These results suggested that maintenance of sufficient left ventricular assist device flow is important in prevention of stroke, which may be related to subclinical pump thrombosis.

COMMENT

Stroke continues to be a major adverse event (AE) following left ventricular assist device (LVAD) implantation. With technological and surgical advances, current generation

*Redrafted abstract

continuous flow pumps have lesser stroke rate compared to the older pulsatile flow pumps. It is the occurrence of such AEs that poses a dilemma for the clinician in choosing the most appropriate therapy—optimal medical management (OMM) versus LVAD.

The eighth INTERMACS annual report (2017) published 10-year data for LVAD implants. Stroke is the leading cause of death following LVAD implantation between 6 months and 4 years of implant occurring at a rate of 2.42 per 100 patient months and 1.12 per 100 patient months within the first 3 months and after 9 months of LVAD implant respectively.

In this study, the authors have analyzed the risk factors for stroke early (within 90 days) after implantation of LVAD. It is a retrospective study looking at 158 patients over 11-year period. Stroke occurred in 28 patients (18%) within 90 days. Of the 28 patients with stroke, 20 patients had hemorrhagic stroke and 8 patients had embolic stroke causing cerebral infarction.

Multivariate analysis in this study revealed perioperative low cardiac output was the only independent risk factor for stroke in the acute phase. They also reported high lactate dehydrogenase (LDH) levels in the early postoperative period which coincided with periods of low cardiac output. The authors hypothesize that low flows (low cardiac output) could lead to subclinical pump thrombosis as suggested by elevations in the LDH levels and cause stroke.

Dr Mark Helmers and Dr Pavan Atluri, in an editorial commentary, pointed out the much higher rates of hemorrhagic stroke (70%) in the study which could not be explained solely by pump thrombosis. Perhaps anticoagulation, acquired von Willebrand syndrome or mycotic aneurysm also played a role in these patients. They concede however, that given higher rates of embolic stroke following LVAD implants in other studies, subclinical pump thrombosis may have a role—though not borne out by data in this study.

This study suggests a possible role of low flows causing subclinical pump thrombosis and one needs to maintain adequate flows in the perioperative period to prevent stagnation and pump thrombosis. Needless to say, we also need to watch out for even brief periods of very high flows and hypertension in an anticoagulated patient—which could also result in a stroke. A balance, therefore, needs to be struck.

ARTICLE 7

Outcomes of Venopulmonary Arterial Extracorporeal Life Support as Temporary Right Ventricular Support after Left Ventricular Assist Implantation

Shehab S, Rao S, Macdonald P, et al. Outcomes of venopulmonary arterial extracorporeal life support as temporary right ventricular support after left ventricular assist implantation.
J Thorac Cardiovasc Surg. 2018;156(6):2143-52.

Abstract*

Objectives: We report our experience with the temporary postoperative venopulmonary arterial extracorporeal life support as short-term right ventricular support among patients who had biventricular failure undergoing HeartWare (HeartWare Inc, Framingham, MA) left ventricular assist device (LVAD) implantation; these outcomes were with isolated LVAD support and long-term biventricular assist device support.

Methods: Total 112 consecutive patients were studied; out of these, 75 patients were with the isolated HeartWare LVAD, 23 patients with concomitant LVAD and venopulmonary arterial extracorporeal life support, and 14 patients were with durable biventricular assist device support. Decision regarding short-term or durable biventricular support was on the basis of clinical characteristics, hemodynamic profile, and echocardiography.

Results: Patients who needed venopulmonary arterial extracorporeal life support following insertion of LVAD needed the greatest support preoperatively and were more likely to have the Interagency Registry for Mechanically Assisted Circulatory Support level 1 (LVAD, 19%; venopulmonary arterial extracorporeal life support, 48%; biventricular assist device, 57%; p <0.001). They were more likely to need preoperative mechanical support (LVAD, 9%; venopulmonary arterial extracorporeal life support, 43%; and biventricular assist device, 29%; p <0.001) or preoperative ventilation (9%, 38%, and 21%, respectively, p <0.05). Preoperative hemodynamic and echocardiographic parameters were more comparable to patients needing isolated LVAD, with patients requiring the durable biventricular assist device support more likely to have increased right atrial pressure (LVAD 14.3 ± 6.7 vs. venopulmonary arterial extracorporeal life support 13.6 ± 4.8 vs. biventricular assist device 18.7 ± 6.0 mm Hg, p <0.05); right atrial/pulmonary capillary wedge pressure ratio (0.53 ± 0.23 vs. 0.51 ± 0.17 vs. 0.69 ± 0.22, respectively, p <0.02); and tricuspid regurgitation grade (1.7 ± 1.5 vs. 1.7 ± 1.6 vs. 2.8 ± 1.6, respectively, p <0.01). One-year survival was 84% for patients who had an isolated LVAD as compared to 62% for patients who had venopulmonary arterial extracorporeal life support and 64.3% for biventricular assist device.

Conclusion: In critically unwell patients who need temporary biventricular support, planned venopulmonary arterial extracorporeal life support gives acceptable outcomes, which are comparable to durable biventricular assist device support. Requirement for the venopulmonary arterial extracorporeal life support is more determined by the level of preoperative acuity as compared to hemodynamic or echocardiographic parameters.

COMMENT

Left ventricular assist devices (LVADs) have shown survival benefits in selected patients with end-stage heart failure (HF) awaiting heart transplantation (HT). Despite technical and surgical advances, implantation of LVAD is associated with right ventricular dysfunction (RVD) in 20–30% of patients. RVD following LVAD dysfunction could

*Redrafted abstract

range in severity from mild-to-moderate and severe levels. Therapy consists of optimizing RV function using pharmacological means, ventilatory adjustments, inhaled nitric oxide and mechanical circulatory support (MCS) in terms of either temporary right ventricular assist device (RVAD) or more durable RVAD—thereby providing biventricular support.

It has also been shown that in cases of moderate-to-severe RVD, timing of instituting RVAD support is crucial with early RVAD support showing superior outcomes compared to patients in whom RVAD was instituted later.

In this study, the authors analyzed 112 patients undergoing LVAD implantation between 2007 and 2016. They consisted of 75 patients with isolated LVAD, 23 patients who required temporary RVAD using venopulmonary arterial extracorporeal life support (VPA-ECLS) and 14 patients with durable RVAD used as biventricular VAD (BiVAD). They reported a 1-year survival of 75% for isolated LVAD, 62% for LVAD with VPA-ECLS and 64.3% for patients with durable biventricular assist device.

The temporary RVAD was established between inflow cannula sited in the right atrium (RA) inserted percutaneously via femoral vein. The outflow cannula was connected and tied securely to an 8-mm Dacron graft sewn onto the main pulmonary artery which was tunneled out of the chest. This technique permitted easy decannulation without having to re-enter the chest in patients who are already very sick. The decision to use VPA-ECLS or BiVAD was based on Echo parameters, RV function and the probability of weaning off RVAD soon.

Right ventricular assist device does not need an oxygenator incorporated if gas exchange by native lung is adequate. Adding an oxygenator increases risk of inflammatory process, coagulopathy and thrombosis.

This study has shown that using extra corporeal membrane oxygenation (ECMO) in a RVAD configuration is as effective as a durable RVAD in the setting of RVD after LVAD implantation.

In our country, where LVAD implantation is not done in very large numbers due to cost involved—this study provides good data showing that temporary ECMO in RVAD configuration can be used as effectively as a durable BiVAD which is much more expensive in those patients who develop severe RVD after LVAD implantation.

ARTICLE 8

Venoarterial Extracorporeal Membrane Oxygenation for Postcardiotomy Shock: Risk Factors for Mortality

Fux T, Holm M, Corbascio M, et al. Venoarterial extracorporeal membrane oxygenation for postcardiotomy shock: Risk factors for mortality.
J Thorac Cardiovasc Surg. 2018;156(5):1894-902.

Abstract*

Objectives: Refractory postcardiotomy cardiogenic shock is related with increased mortality; venoarterial extracorporeal membrane oxygenation provides acute cardiopulmonary life support. This study was aimed at identifying prevenoarterial extracorporeal membrane oxygenation risk factors of 90-day mortality.

Methods: In this study, 105 consecutive patients were retrospectively analyzed; these patients were supported with venoarterial extracorporeal membrane oxygenation because of refractory postcardiotomy cardiogenic shock. Univariable and multivariable logistic regression was used to analyze the association between preimplant variables and all-cause mortality at 90 days.

Results: Main surgical subgroups included single noncoronary artery bypass grafting (29%); isolated coronary artery bypass grafting (20%); and two and three concomitant surgical procedures (31% and 20%, respectively). Median age of patients in study was 62 years (interquartile range, 52–68 years); 76% were males. Cardiopulmonary resuscitation was done in 30% patients before initiation of venoarterial extracorporeal membrane oxygenation. Median duration of venoarterial extracorporeal membrane oxygenation was 7 days (interquartile range, 3–14 days). In-hospital mortality was 56% and 90-day overall mortality was 57%. Out of total patients, 47% of patients died on venoarterial extracorporeal membrane oxygenation, 51% of patients were weaned successfully, 1% patients were bridged to heart transplantation, and 1% patients were bridged to left ventricular assist device. On multivariable logistic regression analysis, arterial lactate [odds ratio (OR) per unit] 1.22, 95% confidence interval (CI) 1.07–14.0, p = 0.004] and ischemic heart disease (OR, 7.87, 95% CI 2.55–24.3, p <0.001) were identified as independent risk factors of 90-day mortality.

Conclusion: In patients who had postcardiotomy cardiogenic shock, ischemic heart disease and the level of arterial lactate before initiation of venoarterial extracorporeal membrane oxygenation were recognized as independent prevenoarterial extracorporeal membrane oxygenation risk factors of 90-day mortality. These risk factors are easily accessible for prevenoarterial extracorporeal membrane oxygenation risk prediction and may also improve selection of patients for this resource-intensive therapy.

COMMENT

Postcardiotomy cardiogenic shock (PCS) is defined as low cardiac output syndrome with evidence of tissue hypoperfusion and end-organ dysfunction in spite of adequate preload; it affects 0.2–6% of patients undergoing cardiothoracic surgery. These patients cannot be weaned off cardiopulmonary bypass machine in the operating theater and are uniformly fatal unless they have other forms of mechanical circulatory support (MCS). Use of MCS in PCS following cardiac surgery has been reported

*Redrafted abstract

as early as 1963. Use of extracorporeal membrane oxygenation (ECMO) in neonates was first reported by Dr Robert Bartlett in 1972.

Use of ECMO gradually increased and became widespread after the publication of the results of CESAR trial in 2009. Venoarterial (VA) ECMO began to be used as a bridge to recovery after PCS in cardiac surgery, as a support in patients undergoing heart and lung transplant. Advances in technology, better understanding of rheology and blood physiology, advances in oxygenators have improved the outcomes of ECMO in recent years. However, among the various indications for ECMO, VA-ECMO for PCS has the worst outcomes with mortality ranging from 60% to 80%.

In this study, the authors have analyzed 105 patients with PCS who were supported by VA-ECMO. Fifty-one percent of these patients were successfully weaned, 47% of these patients died while on VA-ECMO, 1% was bridged to heart transplant and 1% was bridged to durable left ventricular assist device (LVAD). Analysis of various pre-ECMO variables, elevated serum lactate levels and ischemic heart disease were found to be independent risk factors for 90-day mortality.

Serum lactate is a marker for adequacy of tissue perfusion and serial monitoring of lactate levels will guide further management in this subset of extremely sick patients.

While other studies have looked at a combination of pre-ECMO, ECMO and post-ECMO factors, this study is the first one to look only at pre-ECMO variables and outcomes—thereby identifying risk factors which will enable proper selection of PCS cases in which for VA-ECMO would have a good outcome and avoid futile attempts. An elevated serum lactate above 10 mmol/L was associated with high mortality. Similarly, presence of ischemic heart disease had a negative impact on survival. Both these risk factors were found to have similar effects in other studies.

Postcardiotomy cardiogenic shock occurs in about 0.5–1.5% following cardiac surgery and levels of serum lactate can help us deciding appropriate patients who would benefit from VA-ECMO.

INDEX

Page numbers followed *f* refer to figure.